Recent Advances in the Diagnosis and Management of Equine Gastrointestinal Diseases

Editors

HENRY STÄMPFLI
ANGELIKA SCHOSTER

VETERINARY CLINICS OF NORTH AMERICA: EQUINE PRACTICE

www.vetequine.theclinics.com

Consulting Editor
THOMAS J. DIVERS

April 2018 • Volume 34 • Number 1

ELSEVIER

1600 John F. Kennedy Boulevard ● Suite 1800 ● Philadelphia, Pennsylvania, 19103-2899

http://www.vetequine.theclinics.com

VETERINARY CLINICS OF NORTH AMERICA: EQUINE PRACTICE Volume 34, Number 1
April 2018 ISSN 0749-0739, ISBN-13: 978-0-323-58332-9

Editor: Colleen Dietzler
Developmental Editor: Donald Mumford

Veterinary Clinics of North America: Equine Practice (ISSN 0749-0739) is published in April, August, and December by Elsevier Inc., 360 Park Avenue South, New York, NY 10010-1710. Business and Editorial Offices: 1600 John F. Kennedy Blvd., Suite 1800, Philadelphia, PA 19103-2899. Subscription prices are $281.00 per year (domestic individuals), $536.00 per year (domestic institutions), $100.00 per year (domestic students/residents), $328.00 per year (Canadian individuals), $675.00 per year (Canadian institutions), $365.00 per year (international individuals), $675.00 per year (international institutions), and $180.00 per year (international and Canadian students/residents). To receive student/resident rate, orders must be accompanied by name of affiliated institution, date of term, and the signature of program/residency coordinator on institution letterhead. Orders will be billed at individual rate until proof of status is received. Foreign air speed delivery is included in all *Clinics* subscription prices. All prices are subject to change without notice. **POSTMASTER:** Send address changes to *Veterinary Clinics of North America: Equine Practice*, 3251 Riverport Lane, Maryland Heights, MO 63043. Customer Service (orders, claims, online, change of address): Elsevier Health Sciences Division, Subscription **Customer Service, 3251 Riverport Lane, Maryland Heights, MO 63043. Tel: 1-800-654-2452 (U.S. and Canada); 314-447-8871 (outside U.S. and Canada). Fax: 314-447-8029. E-mail: journalscustomerservice-usa@elsevier.com (for print support);** E-mail: **journalsonlinesupport-usa@elsevier. com (for online support).**

Reprints. For copies of 100 or more of articles in this publication, please contact the Commercial Reprints Department, Elsevier Inc., 360 Park Avenue South, New York, NY 10010-1710. Tel.: 212-633-3874; Fax: 212-633-3820; E-mail: reprints@elsevier.com.

Veterinary Clinics of North America: Equine Practice is covered in *MEDLINE/PubMed (Index Medicus), Excerpta Medica, Current Contents/Agriculture, Biology and Environmental Sciences,* and *ISI.*

Contributors

CONSULTING EDITOR

THOMAS J. DIVERS, DVM
Diplomate, American College of Veterinary Internal Medicine; Diplomate, American College of Veterinary Emergency and Critical Care; Steffen Professor of Veterinary Medicine, Section of Large Animal Medicine, College of Veterinary Medicine, Cornell University, Ithaca, New York, USA

EDITORS

HENRY STÄMPFLI, DVM, Dr Med Vet
Diplomate, American College of Veterinary Internal Medicine; Professor, Department of Clinical Studies, Large Animal Medicine, Clinical Studies, Ontario Veterinary College, University of Guelph, Guelph, Ontario, Canada

ANGELIKA SCHOSTER, DVM, Dr Med Vet, PD, DVSc, PhD
Diplomate, American College of Veterinary Internal Medicine; Diplomate, European College of Equine Internal Medicine; Senior Clinical Lecturer, Vetsuisse Faculty, Equine Department, Clinic for Equine Internal Medicine, University of Zurich, Zurich, Switzerland

AUTHORS

FRANK M. ANDREWS, DVM, MS
Diplomate, American College of Veterinary Large Animal Internal Medicine; LVMA Equine Committee Professor and Director, Equine Health Studies Program, Department of Veterinary Clinical Sciences, School of Veterinary Medicine, Louisiana State University, Baton Rouge, Louisiana, USA

LUIS G. ARROYO, Lic. Med. Vet, DVSc, PhD
Diplomate, American College of Veterinary Internal Medicine; Associate Professor, Department of Clinical Studies, Ontario Veterinary College, University of Guelph, Guelph, Ontario, Canada

ANTHONY BLIKSLAGER, DVM, PhD
Diplomate, American College of Veterinary Surgeons; Department of Clinical Sciences, NC State Veterinary Hospital, NC State University, Raleigh, North Carolina, USA

BENJAMIN BUCHANAN, DVM
Diplomate, American College of Veterinary Large Animal Internal Medicine; Diplomate, American College of Veterinary Emergency and Critical Care; Principle Owner and Staff Veterinarian, Brazos Valley Equine Hospitals, Navasota, Texas, USA

MEGAN BURKE, DVM
Diplomate, American College of Veterinary Surgeons; NC State Veterinary Hospital, NC State University, Raleigh, North Carolina, USA

PILAR CAMACHO-LUNA, DVM
Medicine Resident, Equine Health Studies Program, Department of Veterinary Clinical Sciences, School of Veterinary Medicine, Louisiana State University, Baton Rouge, Louisiana, USA

ELIZABETH A. CARR, DVM, PhD
Diplomate, American College of Veterinary Internal Medicine; Diplomate, American College of Veterinary Emergency Critical Care; Associate Chair & Assistant Hospital Director, Department of Large Animal Clinical Sciences, College of Veterinary Medicine, Michigan State University, East Lansing, Michigan, USA

MARCIO CARVALHO COSTA, DVSc, PhD
Department of Veterinary Biomedicine, University of Montreal, Saint-Hyacinthe, Quebec, Canada

NICOLA C. CRIBB, MA, VetMB, DVSc
Diplomate, American College of Veterinary Surgeons; Assistant Professor, Department of Clinical Studies, Ontario Veterinary College, University of Guelph, Guelph, Ontario, Canada

T. ZANE DAVIS, PhD
USDA/ARS Poisonous Plant Research Laboratory, Logan, Utah, USA

C. LANGDON FIELDING, DVM
Diplomate, American College of Veterinary Emergency and Critical Care; Diplomate, American College of Veterinary Sports Medicine and Rehabilitation; Loomis Basin Equine Medical Center, Penryn, California, USA

BRUCE C. McGORUM, BSc, BVM&S, PhD, CEIM, FRCVS
Diplomate, European College of Equine Internal Medicine; Professor of Equine Internal Medicine and Head of Equine Section, Royal (Dick) School of Veterinary Studies, The Roslin Institute, The University of Edinburgh, Roslin, Great Britain

OLIMPO OLIVER-ESPINOSA, DVM, MSc, DVSc
Associate Professor, Department of Animal Health, Faculty of Veterinary Medicine and Zootechnics, National University of Colombia, Bogotá D.C., Colombia

KURT PFISTER, DVM, Dip EVPC
European Parasitology Specialist, Parasite Consulting GmbH, Berne, Switzerland; Institute of Comparative Tropical Medicine and Parasitology, LMU – University Munich, Munich, Germany

R. SCOTT PIRIE, BVM&S, PhD, CEIM, CEP, MRCVS
Diplomate, European College of Equine Internal Medicine; Professor of Equine Clinical Sciences, Royal (Dick) School of Veterinary Studies, The Roslin Institute, The University of Edinburgh, Roslin, Great Britain

ANGELIKA SCHOSTER, DVM, Dr Med Vet, PD, DVSc, PhD
Diplomate, American College of Veterinary Internal Medicine; Diplomate, European College of Equine Internal Medicine; Senior Clinical Lecturer, Vetsuisse Faculty, Equine Department, Clinic for Equine Internal Medicine, University of Zurich, Zurich, Switzerland

SARAH D. SHAW, DVM
Diplomate ACVIM-LA; Associate, Rotenberg Veterinary P.C., Palgrave, Adjunct Professor, Department of Clinical Studies, Ontario Veterinary College, University of Guelph, Guelph, Ontario, Canada

HENRY STÄMPFLI, DVM, Dr Med Vet
Diplomate, American College of Veterinary Internal Medicine; Professor, Department of Clinical Studies, Large Animal Medicine, Clinical Studies, Ontario Veterinary College, University of Guelph, Guelph, Ontario, Canada

BRYAN L. STEGELMEIER, DVM, PhD
USDA/ARS Poisonous Plant Research Laboratory, Logan, Utah, USA

DEBORAH VAN DOORN, DVM, PhD
Department of Infectious Diseases and Immunology, Faculty of Veterinary Medicine, Utrecht University, Utrecht, The Netherlands

JEFFREY SCOTT WEESE, DVSc
Department of Pathobiology, University of Guelph, Guelph, Ontario, Canada

Contents

This article provides readers with the basic concepts necessary to understand studies using recent molecular methods performed in intestinal microbiome assessment, with special emphasis on the high-throughput sequencing. This article also summarizes the current knowledge on this topic and discusses future insights on the interaction between the intestinal microbiome and equine health.

Probiotics are commonly used in human and veterinary medicine owing to their postulated positive effects on overall and specifically gastrointestinal health. Although some beneficial effects have been shown in several human diseases, a general beneficial effect of probiotics is currently not supported. In horses, well-designed studies to date are few, results are conflicting, and the effects of probiotics are questionable. Adverse effects are rare; however, intestinal adverse effects (diarrhea) have been reported in foals. Quality control of over-the-counter probiotics is not tightly regulated, and labels often do not reflect the content.

Diagnostic ultrasonography has been used as a test to determine the presence or absence of gastrointestinal disease in horses and foals. General techniques and anatomic landmarks are reviewed. Many clinical reports that have included diagnostic ultrasound as part of their diagnostic process and accuracy studies are necessary to determine the usefulness of diagnostic ultrasound in clinical practice.

Acute infectious diarrhea in adult horses is a major cause of morbidity and is associated with numerous complications. Common causes include salmonellosis, clostridiosis, Coronavirus infection, and infection with *Neorickettsia risticii* (Potomac horse fever). Treatment is empirical and supportive until results of specific diagnostic tests are available.

Supportive care is aimed at restoring hydration, correcting electrolyte imbalances, and limiting the systemic inflammatory response. The mainstays of therapy are intravenous fluid therapy, electrolyte supplementation where necessary, nonsteroidal antiinflammatory agents, and nutritional support. Specific therapies include colloid oncotic support, antibiotics, hyperimmune plasma, polymyxin B, pentoxifylline, probiotics, binding agents, gastroprotectants, laminitis prevention, and coagulation prophylaxis.

Olimpo Oliver-Espinosa

Diarrhea is one of the most important diseases in young foals and may occur in more than half of foals until weaning age. Several infectious and noninfectious underlying causes have been implicated but scientific evidence of pathogenesis is evolving. It is important to investigate all known potential causes and identify infectious agents to avoid outbreaks, evaluate the level of systemic compromise, and establish adequate therapy. It is crucial to differentiate foals that can be managed in field conditions from those that should be sent to a referral center. This article reviews these aspects and recent developments in the diagnostic and therapeutic approaches.

Olimpo Oliver-Espinosa

Chronic diarrhea in the horse is defined as diarrhea present for more than several days with little if any improvement. The diagnosis and treatment of horses with chronic diarrhea usually present a great challenge to the clinician. There are many limitations to treatment of these patients given the limited numbers in which a final diagnosis can be achieved. The lack of knowledge of the alterations of horse microbiota during chronic diarrhea and the multiplicity of causes also make treatment challenging. A poor prognosis is often attached to chronic diarrhea, particularly in cases with neoplasia and inflammatory bowel disease.

Megan Burke and Anthony Blikslager

Differentiating between medical and surgical causes of colic is one of the primary goals of the colic workup, because early surgical intervention improves prognosis in horses requiring surgery. Despite the increasing availability of advanced diagnostics (hematologic analyses, abdominal ultrasound imaging, etc), the most accurate indicators of the need for surgery remain the presence of moderate to severe signs of abdominal pain, recurrence of pain after appropriate analgesic therapy, and the absence of intestinal borborygmi. Investigation of novel biomarkers, which may help to differentiate surgical lesions from those that can be managed medically, continues to be an active area of research.

Equine gastric ulcer syndrome (EGUS) primarily describes ulceration in the terminal esophagus, nonglandular squamous mucosa, glandular mucosa of the stomach, and proximal duodenum. EGUS is common in all breeds and ages of horses and foals. This article focuses on the current terminology for EGUS, etiologies and pathogenesis for lesions in the nonglandular and glandular stomach, diagnosis, and a comprehensive approach to the treatment and prevention of EGUS in adult horses and foals.

Equine dysautonomia (ED; also known as equine grass sickness) is a neurologic disease of unknown cause, which primarily affects grazing adult horses. The clinical signs reflect degeneration of specific neuronal populations, predominantly within the autonomic and enteric nervous systems, with disease severity and prognosis determined by the extent of neuronal loss. This article is primarily focused on the major clinical decision-making processes in relation to ED, namely, (1) clinical diagnosis, (2) selection of appropriate ancillary diagnostic tests, (3) obtaining diagnostic confirmation, (4) selection of treatment candidates, and (5) identifying appropriate criteria for euthanasia.

Because most poisonings occur by toxin ingestion, the gastrointestinal system is the first exposed and, in most cases, it is exposed to the highest toxin concentrations. Consequently, enterocyte damage is common. However, because many toxins produce organ-specific damage, and enterocyte necrosis is easily confused with autolysis, many gastrointestinal lesions are overlooked or overshadowed by other clinical and pathologic changes. The objective of this work is to review several common toxins and poisonous plants that produce primarily gastrointestinal disease.

Regular anthelmintic treatment has contributed to anthelmintic resistance in horse helminths. This mass anthelmintic treatment was originally developed owing to a lack of larvicidal drugs against *Strongylus vulgaris*. The high prevalence of anthelmintic resistance and shortening of strongyle egg reappearance period after avermectins/moxidectins requires epidemiologically appropriate and sustainable measures. Selective anthelmintic treatment is a much-needed deworming approach: more than 50% of adult horses manifest no strongyle egg excretion. In this article, selective anthelmintic treatment procedure is described, with the specific focus on the advantages of an evidence-based, medically appropriate, and

With advances in technology and owner education, field management in equine veterinary medicine continues to evolve. Equine gastrointestinal disease is one of the most common types of emergencies evaluated by equine practitioners, and many of these patients can be effectively managed in the field. Although the equine veterinarian must make numerous decisions, fluid therapy, pain management, and antimicrobial use are 3 of the major choices that must be addressed when initiating field treatment of equine gastrointestinal disease. This article addresses the practical use of these 3 treatment categories that are essential to field practice.

Nutritional support is an important adjunct to medical therapy in the sick, injured, or debilitated equine patient. What is not clear is the optimal route, composition, or amounts of support. The enteral route should be chosen whenever possible to maximize the benefits to the gastrointestinal tract and the patient as a whole. Complete or partial parenteral nutrition is most useful as a bridge during recovery and transition to enteral feeding in the horse. The reader is encouraged to consider nutritional support whether enteral or parenteral in any anorexic, chronically debilitated, or sick equine patient.

VETERINARY CLINICS OF
NORTH AMERICA: EQUINE PRACTICE

THE CLINICS ARE NOW AVAILABLE ONLINE!
Access your subscription at:
www.theclinics.com

Preface

Advances in the Diagnosis and Management of Equine Gastrointestinal Diseases

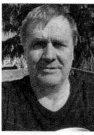 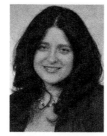

Henry Stämpfli, DVM, Dr Med Vet   Angelika Schoster, DVM, Dr Med Vet, PD, DVSc, PhD

Editors

An illustrious group of colleagues has agreed to commit to writing articles for this issue of *Veterinary Clinics of North America: Equine Practice.* We are very thankful for the excellent work presented here and honored to be the editors. With recent advantages of real-time polymerase chain reaction and next-generation sequencing, a whole new area of research on diagnostic and therapeutic approaches to equine gastrointestinal diseases has opened up for the veterinarian working in practice. In addition, "diagnostic tools" originally developed mostly for referral hospitals are continuously improving, getting smaller, more powerful, and more perfectly suited for the practitioner working in the field. We hope the present issue on gastrointestinal diseases should assist in taking our care for the horse and its owner to the next level.

Henry Stämpfli, DVM, Dr Med Vet
Clinical Studies
Ontario Veterinary College
University of Guelph
50 Stone Road East
Guelph N1G 2W1, Ontario, Canada

Angelika Schoster, DVM, Dr Med Vet, PD, DVSc, PhD
Equine Department
Clinic for Equine Internal Medicine
University of Zurich
Zurich 8057, Switzerland

E-mail addresses:
hstaempf@uoguelph.ca (H. Stämpfli)
aschoster@vetclinics.uzh.ch (A. Schoster)

Vet Clin Equine 34 (2018) xiii
https://doi.org/10.1016/j.cveq.2018.01.001
0749-0739/18/© 2018 Published by Elsevier Inc.

vetequine.theclinics.com

Understanding the Intestinal Microbiome in Health and Disease

Marcio Carvalho Costa, DVSc, PhD[a],*, Jeffrey Scott Weese, DVSc[b]

KEYWORDS

- Intestinal microbiota • Next-generation sequencing • 16S rRNA • Equine • Horse

KEY POINTS

- New technologies have allowed a better understanding of the equine intestinal microbiota and how it interacts with the host.
- The intestinal microbiome is now considered essential for the maintenance of health. Disturbances of this complex ecosystem are associated with several diseases.
- There is abundant interindividual variation in the microbiome and it can be influenced by a range of factors, such as diet, management, and antimicrobial exposure.
- Changes in the intestinal microbiome of horses have been associated with various clinical conditions, including colitis, laminitis, and colic.

INTRODUCTION

The intestinal tract contains a complex polymicrobial community that consists of viruses, archaea, fungi, parasites, and bacteria. The bacterial community is the most extensively studied and is thought to be the most important in maintaining the homeostasis of this complex environment. Overall, the members of this microbial community (the microbiota) and the genetic composition of these microbes (the microbiome) dwarf that of the host. It has been estimated that only 10% to 50% of the human body consists of human cells; within that, human genes only make up 1% (or less) of the overall gene content.[1] Only recently, with high throughput and cost-effective DNA-sequencing technologies, has this area been explored in depth.[1,2] Recent study of these complex microbial communities and their interactions with the host have shown that gut bacteria cause or contribute to the occurrence of conditions such as allergies, inflammatory bowel diseases, rectal cancer, diabetes, and obesity; they are even able to induce alterations of behavioral and mood status.[3]

[a] Department of Veterinary Biomedicine, University of Montreal, 3200 Rue Sicotte, Saint-Hyacinthe, Quebec J2S 2M2, Canada; [b] Department of Pathobiology, University of Guelph, 50 Stone Road East, Guelph, Ontario N1G 2W1, Canada
* Corresponding author.
E-mail address: marcio.costa@umontreal.ca

Vet Clin Equine 34 (2018) 1–12
https://doi.org/10.1016/j.cveq.2017.11.005
0749-0739/18/© 2017 Elsevier Inc. All rights reserved.

vetequine.theclinics.com

The objectives of this article are to familiarize readers with the new concepts and terms used in this research, to provide the necessary knowledge for a good understanding and interpretation of those studies, and to provide an update on the current knowledge of the intestinal microbiome of horses. This article focuses on recent studies using culture-independent methods, mainly next-generation sequencing (NGS). Another article discussing the characterization the intestinal microbiome of horses can be found in the literature.[4]

Basic Concepts

Understanding of some basic microbial ecology concepts is necessary for proper assessment of data and publications. **Table 1** summarizes the definitions of some of the most used concepts.[5,6]

Studies investigating purely the taxonomic classification of bacterial communities (which bacteria are present) should adopt the term microbiota and, if their overall genetic makeup or functional potential is being investigated (eg, shotgun metagenomics), the term microbiome is the most appropriate.

Changes in beta-diversity are noteworthy and differential changes in membership and structure can allow for some useful inferences. For example, if there is a change in membership but not structure, it implies that changes are most likely from rare members being added or dropped. Conversely, if structure changes and membership remains the same, it implies that there are changes in relative numbers (overgrowth or depletion) of existing members, with little deletion or addition of new taxa.

To illustrate these concepts, consider the number of horse breeds found in a 100 km (62 miles) radius of a specified area. If 5 different breeds, Thoroughbred, Standardbred, Belgian, Dutch Warmblood, and Canadian Horse, are identified during sampling, that constitutes a richness of 5. This is a representation of the community

Table 1 Definition of the main concepts used in microbial ecology	
Microbiota	All microorganisms of a particular environment
Microbiome	All microorganisms along with their genetic material and their interaction with an environment
Alpha diversity	Describes characteristics of individual samples (eg, richness, evenness, and diversity)
Richness	Total number of taxa (eg, species or genera, families, phyla) present in an environment, either through direct measure (observed richness) or through calculations to estimate the true richness that would have been detected if the entire population had been studied (estimated richness) Alpha diversity indices can be described and compared between groups (eg, newborn foals have a richer microbiota than older animals)[7]
Evenness	Distribution of species (eg, prevalence or relative abundance of each population within a community)
Diversity	Mathematical equation that takes into account richness and evenness (ie, it quantifies how equal a microbial community is)
Beta-diversity	Comparisons between samples or groups assessed in a variety of ways with different indices Compares the overall composition of the microbiota, typically based on membership or community structure
Membership	Members (eg, species) that are or are not present
Structure	Broader comparison that takes into account the members that are or are not present, and their relative abundance

membership. Now, take into account the distribution of each breed in that same area to find that the population of Thoroughbreds represent 80% of all horses and that Standardbreds are 10%, Dutch Warmblood are 5%, Canadian horses are 4%, and Belgians only 1% (**Fig. 1**). The diversity of this community can be calculated by applying these data to different mathematical formulas (eg, Simpson's index). These are alpha diversity assessments that evaluate a single population or sample. If sampling is performed in a variety of different regions in the same manner, these alpha diversity indices can be compared.

If there is a desire to assess the entire horse population in a region, or more broadly (eg, state, province), more samples or a larger sample size can be taken to better estimate the population. If all horses can be accounted for, that is the absolute richness. This is similar to microbiota assessment, in which these indices allow for estimates that are influenced by sample size and how representative the sample population is compared with the overall studied population. Counting each horse allows for description of the absolute abundance (number) and relative abundance (percentage). Because determination of absolute abundance is not practical (or feasible, in the context of microbiota assessment), description of the individual members is based on relative abundance (percentage).

In the previous horse-breed context, beta-diversity comparison might involve comparison of horse populations in eastern and western US states. Likely, the community membership (the different breeds that are present) is similar, so there is no remarkable difference between regions. However, the relative numbers of these breeds might differ greatly (eg, much higher proportion of quarter horses in the western region), resulting in a significant difference in community structure. Modeling techniques can also be applied to the data to identify differences in groups or evaluate the degree of difference between groups.

Assessment of Microbial Communities

As in other species, characterization of the equine intestinal microbiota began with culture-based methods; however, it was understood that this provided, at best, a

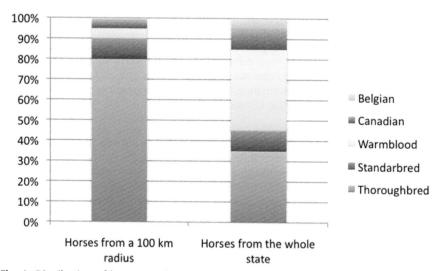

Fig. 1. Distribution of horse populations within 2 different communities. The richness between the communities is the same but they have different diversities.

superficial overview of the microbiota. A large percentage of bacteria are difficult to impossible to culture using routine techniques, and ready growth of some bacteria results in overestimation of their relative abundance.

Development of various culture-independent methods advanced knowledge, but development and widespread accessibility of NGS has been the event that revolutionized understanding of microbiota and the microbiome.

A pool of bacterial genes present in an environment can be sequenced to create metabolic profiles (metagenomic analysis). Although that is a good measure of the genetic capacity of a bacterial community (what they are able to do), it does not necessarily mean they are expressing those genes.

Messenger RNA (metatranscriptomics) and protein (metaproteomics) analyses can be used as indicators of gene expression but, currently, at substantial cost, and instability of the material and database quality are some of the limiting factors for a broader use of those techniques.

Finally, many potential aspects of microbial growth and activity can be assessed by analyzing bacterial byproducts (metabolomics, proteomics).

THE INTESTINAL MICROBIOME
Importance of the Intestinal Microbiome

The intestinal microbiome has long been recognized for its importance in the breakdown of complex food particles, protection against overgrowth of pathogenic organisms, development of the intestinal epithelium, and modulation of the local immune system and metabolic functions. Recently, the intestinal microbiota has also been implicated in actively participating in the pathophysiology of several diseases,[3] including many distant from the gastrointestinal tract.

The Equine Intestinal Microbiome

The large intestine of the horse is an anaerobic chamber where short-chain fatty acids are produced by fibrolytic bacteria through fermentation of complex carbohydrates, supplying most of the horse's energy needs.[8,9] Horses are evolutionarily adapted for grazing with a continuous intake of low amounts of roughage (browsing). However, supplementation with readily digestible carbohydrate has become necessary for horses performing high-energy needs activities. Consequently, diseases affecting the gastrointestinal system are among the main causes of mortality in this species, with particular risk in horses fed high-concentrate diets that diverge from the evolutionary basic.[10] A properly functioning intestinal tract and intestinal microbiota are critical for maintenance of health and performance, but minor stressing factors can lead to imbalances that can have catastrophic consequences.[11]

The intestinal microbiota of healthy horses

It is important to have an understanding of the normal microbiota to enable assessment of abnormal. However, what truly constitutes normal is elusive because there can be marked interhorse variation and a plethora of factors can influence the composition of the microbiota in healthy horses. Normal may vary between regions, ages, management systems, and potentially even breeds; therefore, broad assessment of populations is required to have any understanding of normal.

Consistent with most other mammalian species, Firmicutes is the main bacterial phylum found in the distal gut of horses (**Fig. 2**). There is some inconsistency in the literature, with studies showing Bacteroidetes as the second most abundant phylum,[9,12–15] with others pointing toward Verrucomicrobia.[16–19] Assessment of phyla provides a very high-level overview of the microbiota, and concurrent description of

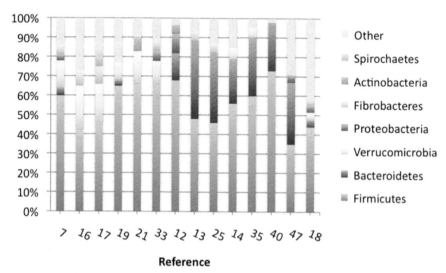

Reference

Fig. 2. Relative abundance of the main Phyla reported in feces of healthy horses.

lower taxonomic levels is required. In general, a few classes, orders, families, and genera predominate in healthy horses.

One important and consistent finding with the use of NGS is recognition that bacteria from the class Clostridia (as well as several *Clostridium* spp) account for most species present in the distal intestinal tract of horses. In the past, this group of bacteria was consistently associated with pathogenicity, but many are currently recognized as commensal and even used for restoration of altered microbiomes.[20] In addition, as in other species, members of the Lachnospiraceae family (within the order Clostridiales and the class Clostridia) also seem to be depleted in sick horses and its role in maintenance of health deserves further investigation.[12,21]

The intestinal colonization of foals

The colonization of the intestinal tract starts with the contact of the foal with the mother's vaginal microbiota and subsequent exposure to other microbial sites on the mare (eg, skin of the udder) and the general environment. Over the next few days, several species will try to establish residence in this highly competitive environment that has the ideal conditions for growth of most bacteria. Therefore, perhaps counterintuitively, newborn foals possess a richer, more diverse, and highly dynamic microbiota compared with older animals[7,15,22,23] (**Fig. 3**).

Several factors seem to determine which bacterial species will colonize the intestinal tract of the newborn. Marked changes in composition and structure of intestinal bacteria have been observed in mares during late gestation compared with a control group,[21] with similar results reported in women.[24] Those are changes that can affect the newborn because the maternal intestinal tract and perineum are a leading source of bacterial exposure during parturition and early life, especially considering the coprophagic habits of foals.

After colonization by the pioneer bacteria, the microbiota present during the first month of life is quite distinct (see **Fig. 3**), which may be related to the influence of colostrum, milk, coprophagy, and the introduction of fiber and, in some cases, carbohydrates to the diet. Yet, controlled studies investigating the impact of each of those factors remain to be performed. The intestinal microbiota becomes stable and more

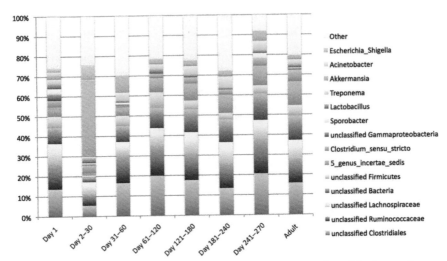

Fig. 3. Relative abundance (%) of the main bacterial genera found in feces of mares and foals at different age groups. (*From* Costa MC, Stampfli HR, Allen-Vercoe E, et al. Development of the fecal microbiota in foals. Equine Vet J 2016;48(6):684; with permission.)

similar to that found in adults after 60 days of life.[7] As in humans, older horses (19–28 years) displayed higher diversity compared with adult animals (5–12 years).[25]

After weaning, marked changes in bacterial communities occur, which might be related to stress.[26] Furthermore, different intestinal microbiota patters (enterotypes) seemed to have different adaptation response to stress.

Finally, the relationship between bacterial colonization and the immune system and the development of immune-related conditions, such as inflammatory airway disease, recurrent airway obstruction, and inflammatory bowel diseases, also remains purely speculative in horses.

Differences in the microbiota throughout the gastrointestinal tract
Studies of the equine intestinal microbiota typically evaluate feces because it is the only component of gastrointestinal tract contents that is easily and noninvasively accessible. The gastrointestinal tract is far from homogenous and factors such as pH, enzymatic digestion, and oxygen tension vary greatly throughout its length. Not surprisingly, significant differences have been reported in bacterial structures present at the different intestinal sites of horses.[13,17,27,28] Fecal samples are representative of the microbiota present in the large colon and, therefore, may be used to detect microbial dysbiosis in the distal gut of horses[13,17,28]; however, the relationship between feces and more proximal regions declines and feces are a poor indicator of the composition of the small intestine.

Factors affecting the intestinal microbiota of horses
As in other species, several conditions can induce changes in the microbial membership and structure of horses, especially at lower taxonomic levels (eg, genus and species). Factors affecting the intestinal microbiota include age, diet, environmental conditions (eg, geographic location, climate, hygiene, fasting, transportation, exercise), inflammation, and the use of external compounds, such as prebiotics, probiotics and antibiotics.[20,29–36]

Diet and management After birth, diet seems to be the most important factor modulating humans' intestinal microbiota.[37] Differences in composition and higher diversity have been shown in the intestines of babies receiving formula compared with mother's milk,[38] but the impact of milk replacers in foals has not been investigated.

As expected, the most marked differences reported in horses are between those on forage-based diets versus carbohydrate supplemented animals.[25,39–41] Indeed, the comparison of the intestinal microbiota of 6 healthy horses revealed marked similarities between the 2 housed in neighboring stalls and those kept outside.[12]

Interestingly, changes at the phylum level (increased Fibrobacteres) have been reported after weaning,[7] but further studies are necessary for a better understanding of this practice in foals.

Several changes in the intestinal microbiota have also been reported after supplementation with prebiotics,[42,43] but the ability of probiotics to induce permanent changes in the gut microbiota is questionable.[35]

Consequences of antibiotic therapy on the intestinal microbiota Among all external factors leading to microbiota changes, administration of antimicrobial drugs may have the most profound consequences.[44] Although antimicrobials are among the most important therapies in horses, they are also associated antimicrobial-associated colitis, something that is presumed to occur following disruption of the resident commensal bacterial community (dysbiosis), allowing colonization or overgrowth by naturally resistant pathogenic organisms (eg, *Clostridium difficile*).[11,45–47] One study demonstrated specific changes in community membership and structure after 5 days of treatment according to the antibiotic administered.[16] Trimethoprim sulfonamide had the most marked effect on the microbiota of horses (compared with penicillin and ceftiofur). However, it was also the only drug administered orally, and it is unclear whether this was because of a greater inherent impact of the drug or because of the route of administration. Nevertheless, the intestinal microbial community of healthy adult horses seems to be resilient because most changes caused by antibiotics were inapparent or minimized 30 days after treatment.[16,48]

Other consequences of the microbial changes due to the use of antibiotics in horses, such as increased incidence of allergic diseases in children,[49] respiratory allergic disease,[50] and increased adiposity,[51] have not been investigated.

Other Several other factors are likely to induce changes in the intestinal microbiota of horses but, as previously indicated, this field of study in this species is only beginning. To date, stressing factors, such as fasting, transportation,[30,34] late pregnancy,[21] and extreme exercise,[33] have been suggested.

Diseases Associated with an Altered Intestinal Microbiota

Several diseases are likely to be associated with changes in the intestinal microbiota of horses, but the differentiation of cause versus effect can be quite difficult. Studies evaluating the microbiota before, during, and after disease can help answer important questions about causality but are very difficult to perform with sporadic diseases. Thus, although it is useful to determine differences that occur in diseased individuals compared with healthy controls, it is important to remember that these often can only be considered differences, not causal events.

Colitis

Despite the high mortality rates and the economic importance of colitis in horses, this disease has not been extensively investigated. As it has been shown in other species, horses with colitis generally present very distinct patters of bacterial communities compared with healthy animals.[12,36] The role of less usual pathogenic bacteria causative of diarrhea is another topic that deserves better attention because most cases still remain undiagnosed. In part, this may be related to poor diagnostic efforts because only the main causes of colitis in horses are normally investigated (eg, C difficile, Clostridium perfringens, Salmonella spp, Neorickettsia risticii). For instance, other organisms, such as Fusobacterium spp and Escherichia spp, have been found in diarrheic horses but not in healthy animals,[12,36] but it is difficult to make conclusions based on those limited descriptive studies and to determine whether these organisms are there because they are causing disease or whether they have been able to colonize and proliferate in response to the altered microbiota from disease.

Nevertheless, decreased richness has been reported in patients with diarrhea and the phylum Firmicutes seems to be depleted in horses with colitis. As in other species, the role of members of the Lachnospiraceae family might be key to the maintenance of the intestinal homeostasis[12,21,36] and future trials may confirm this hypothesis.

Laminitis

The impact of carbohydrate overload in the intestinal microbiota of horses developing laminitis is well established.[52] Recently, molecular methods have been used to better characterize changes after supplementation with short-chain fructooligosaccharides, identifying proliferation of Streptococcus spp in the distal gut of horses before the onset of laminitis and the increase of lactobacilli and Escherichia coli after the onset of the disease.[43,52–54]

One study using NGS suggested a link between specific alterations of the intestinal microbiota and chronic laminitis, but this is more likely to be related to the stress caused by chronic pain stimulation.[19]

Colic

Considering that the intestinal microbiota is quite sensitive to so many stressors, it is expected that marked changes will occur after episodes of colic, even though the cause and severity may be very different in each case.

Again, despite of the importance of this condition, few studies have been performed evaluating the consequences of colic to the intestinal microbiota of horses, reporting increases in bacteria from Bacteroidetes[55] and Proteobacteria[21] compared with non-colic animals. Interestingly, a study also reported consistent changes in certain bacterial taxa before the onset of large colon volvulus,[21] supporting a causative role and suggesting that monitoring of the fecal microbiota might be used as a diagnostic tool for early detection and treatment of certain colic episodes in horses. In addition, various groups were associated with increased risk of colic and Lachnospiraceae and Ruminococcaceae being associated with healthy controls, which emphasizes the importance of these groups. Although it is not adequate to establish a relationship, those changes were more likely a consequence rather than a cause of colic.

Other

Specific alterations in microbial populations have been reported in horses suffering from equine grass sickness, such as greater number of clostridial species (with a lower number of total clostridial counts) in the ileum.[56] More detailed changes in horses suffering from this condition are currently under investigation and include increases in Desulfovibrio and Veillonella spp.[57]

Horses with metabolic syndrome have also been shown to carry a less diverse fecal microbiota with altered community structure compared with controls.[58] A member of subdivision 5 of Verrucomicrobia was associated with animals with the syndrome, whereas Fibrobacter was representative of controls.

FUTURE DIRECTIONS

Based on the recent advances in the characterization of the intestinal microbiota of horses, microbiota manipulation will likely be used in the near future for prevention and treatment of diseases, to diagnose conditions causing or caused by microbial dysbiosis, and to enhance animal performance.

Microbiota manipulation can be achieved by controlling diet, nutrients, and supplements, such as prebiotics, or by using therapies, such as antibiotics, probiotics, and bacteriophages. Alternatively, the whole ecosystem can be transferred to another individual by enema or orally. This procedure, also called fecal microbiota transplantation (FMT) consists of transferring feces (or colonic content) from a healthy individual (donor) to a patient with diarrhea or some other disease state. This has been used with great success in humans for the restoration of the normal microbiota in cases of recurrent *C difficile* infection[59] and it has been used in horses empirically for a long time.[60]

A protocol to perform FMT in horses with diarrhea has been suggested.[61] However, the efficiency of the procedure might be lower in this species due to the anatomic location of the large colon. The transplanted content cannot reach the large colon when delivered by enema because of the long size of the small colon. Furthermore, if the content is delivered by nasogastric tube, the low pH from the stomach, along with digestive enzymes from the proximal intestinal tract, could decrease the efficiency of the procedure.[59] Therefore, controlled studies evaluating adaptations of the procedure for horses are required to better identify conditions that might be responsive to FMT, along with optimal donors, donor screening methods, and administration methods (eg, dose, frequency, whether pretreatment to suppress gastric acid is required).

Synthetic products containing several bacterial species (including some *Clostridium* spp) have been developed for use in humans[20] to provide a stable, reproducible, quality-controlled, and pathogen-free treatment. However, the development of products specifically designed for the equine species might be necessary for the treatment and prevention of colitis in horses.

Microbial manipulation may also be used to prevent or minimize signs of foal heat diarrhea, in which an early and more gradual adaptation of the microbiota may be achieved. However, a better understanding of the microbial changes occurring during this period of the foal's life is required.

Finally, the use of microbiota manipulation to improve animal health is a promising and ongoing field of research. In the near future, it will likely be used for diet adaptation, improvement of animal performance, and to identify specific interactions between intestinal bacteria and the immune system that may enhance protection against infectious diseases.

REFERENCES

1. Sender R, Fuchs S, Milo R. Are we really vastly outnumbered? Revisiting the ratio of bacterial to host cells in humans. Cell 2016;164(3):337–40.
2. Eckburg PB, Bik EM, Bernstein CN, et al. Diversity of the human intestinal microbial flora. Science 2005;308(5728):1635–8.
3. Goulet O. Potential role of the intestinal microbiota in programming health and disease. Nutr Rev 2015;73(Suppl 1):32–40.
4. Costa MC, Weese JS. The equine intestinal microbiome. Anim Health Res Rev 2012;13(1):121–8.
5. Marchesi JR, Ravel J. The vocabulary of microbiome research: a proposal. Microbiome 2015;3:31.

6. Chao A. Nonparametric estimation of the number of classes in a population. Scand J Stat 1984;11(4). https://doi.org/10.2307/4615964.

7. Costa MC, Stampfli HR, Allen-Vercoe E, et al. Development of the faecal microbiota in foals. Equine Vet J 2016;48(6):681–8.

8. Argenzio RA, Southworth M, Stevens CE. Sites of organic acid production and absorption in the equine gastrointestinal tract. Am J Physiol 1974;226(5):1043–50.

9. Daly K, Stewart CS, Flint HJ, et al. Bacterial diversity within the equine large intestine as revealed by molecular analysis of cloned 16S rRNA genes. FEMS Microbiol Ecol 2001;38(2–3):141–51.

10. Al Jassim RA, Andrews FM. The bacterial community of the horse gastrointestinal tract and its relation to fermentative acidosis, laminitis, colic, and stomach ulcers. Vet Clin North Am Equine Pract 2009;25(2):199–215.

11. Cohen ND, Woods AM. Characteristics and risk factors for failure of horses with acute diarrhea to survive: 122 cases (1990-1996). J Am Vet Med Assoc 1999;214(3):382–90.

12. Costa MC, Arroyo LG, Allen-Vercoe E, et al. Comparison of the fecal microbiota of healthy horses and horses with colitis by high throughput sequencing of the V3-V5 region of the 16S rRNA gene. PLoS One 2012;7(7):e41484.

13. Dougal K, la Fuente de G, Harris PA, et al. Identification of a core bacterial community within the large intestine of the horse. PLoS One 2013;8(10):e77660.

14. O'Donnell MM, Harris HMB, Jeffery IB, et al. The core faecal bacterial microbiome of Irish Thoroughbred racehorses. Lett Appl Microbiol 2013;57(6):492–501.

15. Whitfield-Cargile CM, Cohen ND, Suchodolski J, et al. Composition and diversity of the fecal microbiome and inferred fecal metagenome does not predict subsequent pneumonia caused by *Rhodococcus equi* in foals. PLoS One 2015;10(8):e0136586.

16. Costa MC, Stampfli HR, Arroyo LG, et al. Changes in the equine fecal microbiota associated with the use of systemic antimicrobial drugs. BMC Vet Res 2015;11:19.

17. Costa MC, Silva G, Ramos RV, et al. Characterization and comparison of the bacterial microbiota in different gastrointestinal tract compartments in horses. Vet J 2015;205(1):74–80.

18. Shepherd ML, Swecker WSJ, Jensen RV, et al. Characterization of the fecal bacteria communities of forage-fed horses by pyrosequencing of 16S rRNA V4 gene amplicons. FEMS Microbiol Lett 2012;326(1):62–8.

19. Steelman SM, Chowdhary BP, Dowd S, et al. Pyrosequencing of 16S rRNA genes in fecal samples reveals high diversity of hindgut microflora in horses and potential links to chronic laminitis. BMC Vet Res 2012;8(1). https://doi.org/10.1186/1746-6148-8-231.

20. Petrof EO, Gloor GB, Vanner SJ, et al. Stool substitute transplant therapy for the eradication of *Clostridium difficile* infection: "RePOOPulating" the gut. Microbiome 2013;1(1):3.

21. Weese JS, Holcombe SJ, Embertson RM, et al. Changes in the faecal microbiota of mares precede the development of post partum colic. Equine Vet J 2015;47(6):641–9.

22. Bordin AI, Suchodolski JS, Markel ME, et al. Effects of administration of live or inactivated virulent rhodococccus equi and age on the fecal microbiome of neonatal foals. PLoS One 2013;8(6):e66640.

23. Faubladier C, Sadet-Bourgeteau S, Philippeau C, et al. Molecular monitoring of the bacterial community structure in foal feces pre- and post-weaning. Anaerobe 2014;25:61–6.

24. Koren O, Goodrich JK, Cullender TC, et al. Host remodeling of the gut microbiome and metabolic changes during pregnancy. Cell 2012;150(3):470–80.

25. Dougal K, la Fuente de G, Harris PA, et al. Characterisation of the faecal bacterial community in adult and elderly horses fed a high fibre, high oil or high starch diet using 454 pyrosequencing. PLoS One 2014;9(2):e87424.

26. Mach N, Foury A, Kittelmann S, et al. The effects of weaning methods on gut microbiota composition and horse physiology. Front Physiol 2017;8:535.

27. Schoster A, Arroyo LG, Staempfli HR, et al. Comparison of microbial populations in the small intestine, large intestine and feces of healthy horses using terminal restriction fragment length polymorphism. BMC Res Notes 2013;6:91.

28. Ericsson AC, Johnson PJ, Lopes MA, et al. A microbiological map of the healthy equine gastrointestinal tract. PLoS One 2016;11(11):e0166523.

29. Elazab N, Mendy A, Gasana J, et al. Probiotic administration in early life, atopy, and asthma: a meta-analysis of clinical trials. Pediatrics 2013;132(3):e666–76.

30. Faubladier C, Chaucheyras-Durand F, da Veiga L, et al. Effect of transportation on fecal bacterial communities and fermentative activities in horses: impact of *Saccharomyces cerevisiae* CNCM I-1077 supplementation. J Anim Sci 2013; 91(4):1736–44.

31. Perkins GA, Bakker den HC, Burton AJ, et al. Equine stomachs harbor an abundant and diverse mucosal microbiota. Appl Environ Microbiol 2012;78(8): 2522–32.

32. Ladirat SE, Schols HA, Nauta A, et al. High-throughput analysis of the impact of antibiotics on the human intestinal microbiota composition. J Microbiol Methods 2013;92(3):387–97.

33. Almeida MLM, Feringer WHJ, Carvalho JRG, et al. Intense exercise and aerobic conditioning associated with chromium or L-carnitine supplementation modified the fecal microbiota of fillies. PLoS One 2016;11(12):e0167108.

34. Schoster A, Mosing M, Jalali M, et al. Effects of transport, fasting and anaesthesia on the faecal microbiota of healthy adult horses. Equine Vet J 2016;48(5): 595–602.

35. Schoster A, Guardabassi L, Staempfli HR, et al. The longitudinal effect of a multi-strain probiotic on the intestinal bacterial microbiota of neonatal foals. Equine Vet J 2016;48(6):689–96.

36. Rodriguez C, Taminiau B, Brevers B, et al. Faecal microbiota characterisation of horses using 16 rdna barcoded pyrosequencing, and carriage rate of *Clostridium difficile* at hospital admission. BMC Microbiol 2015;15:181.

37. De Filippo C, Cavalieri D, Di Paola M, et al. Impact of diet in shaping gut microbiota revealed by a comparative study in children from Europe and rural Africa. Proc Natl Acad Sci U S A 2010;107(33):14691–6.

38. Azad MB, Konya T, Maughan H, et al. Gut microbiota of healthy Canadian infants: profiles by mode of delivery and infant diet at 4 months. CMAJ 2013;185(5): 385–94.

39. Willing B, Voros A, Roos S, et al. Changes in faecal bacteria associated with concentrate and forage-only diets fed to horses in training. Equine Vet J 2009; 41(9):908–14.

40. Daly K, Proudman CJ, Duncan SH, et al. Alterations in microbiota and fermentation products in equine large intestine in response to dietary variation and intestinal disease. Br J Nutr 2012;107(7):989–95.

41. Fernandes KA, Kittelmann S, Rogers CW, et al. Faecal microbiota of forage-fed horses in New Zealand and the population dynamics of microbial communities following dietary change. PLoS One 2014;9(11):e112846.

42. Respondek F, Goachet AG, Julliand V. Effects of dietary short-chain fructooligo-saccharides on the intestinal microflora of horses subjected to a sudden change in diet. J Anim Sci 2008;86(2):316–23.

43. Milinovich GJ, Burrell PC, Pollitt CC, et al. Microbial ecology of the equine hindgut during oligofructose-induced laminitis. ISME J 2008;2(11):1089–100.

44. Jalanka-Tuovinen J, Salonen A, Nikkilä J, et al. Intestinal microbiota in healthy adults: temporal analysis reveals individual and common core and relation to intestinal symptoms. PLoS One 2011;6(7):e23035.

45. Barr BS, Waldridge BM, Morresey PR, et al. Antimicrobial-associated diarrhoea in three equine referral practices. Equine Vet J 2013;45(2):154–8.

46. Harlow BE, Lawrence LM, Flythe MD. Diarrhea-associated pathogens, lactobacilli and cellulolytic bacteria in equine feces: responses to antibiotic challenge. Vet Microbiol 2013;166(1–2):225–32.

47. Gustafsson A, Baverud V, Gunnarsson A, et al. Study of faecal shedding of *Clostridium difficile* in horses treated with penicillin. Equine Vet J 2004;36(2):180–2.

48. Liepman RS. Alterations in the fecal microbiome of healthy horses in response to antibiotic treatment. Columbia (OH): The Ohio State University; 2015.

49. Floistrup H, Swartz J, Bergstrom A, et al. Allergic disease and sensitization in Steiner school children. J Allergy Clin Immunol 2006;117(1):59–66.

50. Noverr MC, Noggle RM, Toews GB, et al. Role of antibiotics and fungal microbiota in driving pulmonary allergic responses. Infect Immun 2004;72(9):4996–5003.

51. Cho I, Yamanishi S, Cox L, et al. Antibiotics in early life alter the murine colonic microbiome and adiposity. Nature 2012;488(7413):621–6.

52. Garner HE, Moore JN, Johnson JH, et al. Changes in the caecal flora associated with the onset of laminitis. Equine Vet J 1978;10(4):249–52.

53. Crawford C, Sepulveda MF, Elliott J, et al. Dietary fructan carbohydrate increases amine production in the equine large intestine: implications for pasture-associated laminitis. J Anim Sci 2007;85(11):2949–58.

54. Milinovich GJ, Trott DJ, Burrell PC, et al. Changes in equine hindgut bacterial populations during oligofructose-induced laminitis. Environ Microbiol 2006;8(5):885–98.

55. Vanable EB, Kerley MS, Straub R. Assessment of equine fecal microbial profiles during and after a colic episode using pyrosequencing. J Equine Vet Sci 2013;33(5):347–8.

56. Garrett LA, Brown R, Poxton IR. A comparative study of the intestinal microbiota of healthy horses and those suffering from equine grass sickness. Vet Microbiol 2002;87(1):81–8.

57. Leng J, Proudman CJ, Blow F, et al. Understanding intestinal microbiota in equine grass sickness: next generation sequencing of faecal bacterial DNA. Equine Vet J 2015;47(S48):9.

58. Elzinga SE, Weese JS, Adams AA. Comparison of the fecal microbiota in horses with equine metabolic syndrome and metabolically normal controls fed a similar all-forage diet. J Equine Vet Sci 2016;44:9–16.

59. Gough E, Shaikh H, Manges AR. Systematic review of intestinal microbiota transplantation (fecal bacteriotherapy) for recurrent *Clostridium difficile* infection. Clin Infect Dis 2011;53(10):994–1002.

60. McGorum BC, Dixon PM, Smith DG. Use of metronidazole in equine acute idiopathic toxaemic colitis. Vet Rec 1998;142(23):635–8.

61. Muller KR, Yasuda K, Divers TJ, et al. Equine faecal microbiota transplant: current knowledge, proposed guidelines and future directions. Equine Vet Educ 2016. https://doi.org/10.1111/eve.12559.

Probiotic Use in Equine Gastrointestinal Disease

Angelika Schoster, DVM, Dr Med Vet, PD, DVSc, PhD

KEYWORDS

- *Lactobacillus* • *Bifidobacterium* • *Saccharomyces boulardii* • Microbiota
- Fecal microbial transplantation

KEY POINTS

- Mechanisms of action include modulation of the immune system, antimicrobial production, bacterial toxin inactivation, and an increase in colonization resistance.
- Probiotics are generally considered safe, and adverse effects are rare; however, adverse effects have been reported in foals and therefore should be used with caution.
- The quality control of commercial human and veterinary probiotics products is poor and the content of over-the-counter probiotics is often inaccurate regarding bacterial species and amount of live organisms contained in a product.
- The evidence behind efficacy of probiotics in equine gastrointestinal disease is weak and their beneficial effects are questionable.
- Future research on the use of probiotics should focus on using different strains, such as members of families with high abundance in the gastrointestinal system of horses, or a mix of many bacterial strains, similar to fecal microbial transplantation.

INTRODUCTION

Elie Metchnikoff[1] studied the longevity of a group of Bulgarians in the 1900s. He observed that these people ate large amounts of fermented milk and postulated that the bacteria responsible for fermentation had a positive effect on the health of the consumers. These bacteria were named *Lactobacillus bulgaricu*s and the idea of probiotics was born. Metchnikoff initially defined probiotics as "live microorganisms, which exhibit a health promoting effect" in 1908.[1] Although research initially flourished and more probiotic bacterial strains were discovered, it then drifted to the fringe of medical practice and was rediscovered in the mid-1990s. The idea of probiotics exerting beneficial effects has since re-entered the humane medical field and achieved mainstream medical interest. The Food and Agricultural Organization and World Health Organization modified the initial definition to "live microorganisms,

Vetsuisse Faculty, Equine Department, University of Zurich, Winterthurerstrasse 260, Zurich 8057, Switzerland
E-mail address: aschoster@vetclinics.uzh.ch

Vet Clin Equine 34 (2018) 13–24
https://doi.org/10.1016/j.cveq.2017.11.004
0749-0739/18/© 2017 Elsevier Inc. All rights reserved.

that when administered orally at adequate concentrations, provide a beneficial effect beyond that of their nutritional value."[2]

GENERAL CONSIDERATIONS

Information regarding probiotics is accumulating rapidly and is widely available on the Internet and from various sources; thus, it is important to understand some practical aspects regarding formulation and labeling of probiotics that make it challenging to provide direct comparisons and interpret results of studies.

Several microorganisms, including yeasts and bacteria are used as probiotics (**Box 1**). Some bacterial families, mainly lactic acid producers, such as lactobacilli and bifidobacteria, are commonly used. Not all members of the same family have probiotic properties; for example, not all lactobacilli are suitable for probiotic use. Lactobacilli per se are often called probiotics or used as such, but not all lactobacilli have probiotic properties; therefore, the administration of commercial yoghurts is unlikely to be of benefit to the horse. Potential probiotic strains need to be evaluated for suitability of their probiotic characteristics.[3] Potential probiotic strains should be able to survive the gastric environment, have antimicrobial properties, and adhere to mucus and epithelial cells.[2] Not all strains survive the extrusion and drying, which leads to low numbers of active colonies in the end product. The manufacturing process affects the ability of bacteria to maintain desirable traits. Manufacturing a probiotic strain under different conditions, such as varying culture media or coculturing with prebiotics or other probiotic strains, leads to expression of different traits and differences in the final product.[4,5] It is crucial to remember, when comparing results of commercial probiotic

---

Box 1
Bacterial genera and yeasts typically used as probiotics

Saccharomyces (yeast)[a]

Lactobacillus[a]

Bacteroides

Escherichia coli

Enterococcus[a]

Bacillus[a]

Nitrobacter

Nitrosomonas

Streptococcus[a]

Rhodobacter

Fusobacterium

Butyrivibrio

Rhodobacter

Clostridium

Eubacterium

Bifidobacterium[a]

Genera are bacteria unless stated otherwise.
  [a] Evaluated as probiotics in horses.

product studies, that manufacturing methods matter and products containing the same strain at the same concentration cannot be directly compared.

Most diseases of the gastrointestinal tract in horses affect the large intestine. Accordingly, a probiotic used for horses should ideally exert effects in the cecum and colon of horses. Recent advances in research have shown that the most commonly used genera for probiotics, namely *Lactobacillus* spp, *Bifidobacterium* spp, and *Enterococcus* spp are not the most abundant species in the large colon of the hosts. In fact, these species constitute less than 1% of the large intestinal microbiota in healthy horses.[6–8] In horses these bacteria are more abundant in the small compared with the large intestine. In younger animals (less than two months), they are more abundant independently of the gastrointestinal segment; however, still have low abundance when taken into relation with other bacteria.[6,8] The most abundant phylum in the equine gastrointestinal tract is Firmicutes, which contains the class of Clostridia. Important members of the Clostridia class, including *Ruminococcaceae* and *Lachnospiraceae*, have consistently been associated with gastrointestinal health in humans and animals, including horses.[9–11] Lactobacilli and bifidobacteria are not consistently associated with gastrointestinal health and might, therefore, have less influence on the gastrointestinal health of horses. To date, studies investigating effects of members of the Clostridia class are lacking. These might have better effects than currently available probiotic strains.

Studies in healthy animals are often used to assess the ability of a microorganism to survive transit in the gastrointestinal tract and persist after cessation of administration. Effective transit is defined as identification of probiotic microorganisms in fecal material, as determined by bacterial culture or polymerase chain reaction (PCR) assay. Identification of DNA with PCR does not imply viability, rather that a microorganism was present in the probiotic and recognizable DNA sequences survived gastrointestinal passage. Some investigators presume that colonization of the gastrointestinal tract with the probiotic strain is superior to mere effective transit because probiotics could act beyond the period of administration. In vitro studies have revealed, however, that effects of nonviable organism may be greater than the effects of viable organism. Therefore, lack of viability or persistence does not imply lack of effect.

Generally, host-specific strains are believed to be able to colonize the gastrointestinal tract of the indigenous host for longer periods of time. Colonization of the adult equine gastrointestinal tract with *Lactobacillus rhamnosus* LGG of human origin was shown to be poor.[12] After a 5-day course of probiotic administration at 3 different dosages (1 × 10^9, 1 × 10^10, and 5 × 10^10 colony-forming units [CFUs]/g), fecal recovery in 21 adults was shown to be 71%, 29%, and 86% after 24 hours for each dose, respectively. After 48 hours, the probiotic was recovered from the feces of 14%, 14%, and 56% of the total dose administered, respectively, whereas 3 days after administration only one horse in each of the lower two dosage groups remained positive. Fecal recovery was longer in foals, where the probiotic could be recovered up to nine days after administration in some foals.[12] This suggests that the immature gastrointestinal flora of foals could facilitate probiotic survival.

As described previously, foals and adults showed a lack of dose response, making it difficult to determine an ideal dose to use.[12] Similar results were obtained when administering *Saccharomyces boulardii*.[13] After administration of 10 × 10^9 CFUs/g to 3 horses and 20 × 10^9 CFUs/g to 2 horses for 10 days, fecal samples were negative for *S boulardii* on day 20. On day five, all horses had viable *S boulardii* in their feces.[13] Similarly, *S cerevisiae* has been shown to survive but not colonize the ceca and colons of horses.[14–16] This indicates that any beneficial effect of probiotics might not continue beyond the period of administration, making long-term or repeated treatment a necessity.

To assess the effect of probiotics on the composition of the gastrointestinal microbiota, reduction of pathogens in vivo studies, in particular, have been conducted in other animal species. Knowledge regarding composition and function of the microbiota is not fully understood. For example, enteric pathogens, such as *Clostridium difficile* and *Salmonella*, can be isolated from feces of healthy animals[17]; therefore, presence of presumed pathogenic organisms does not necessarily cause disease and any attempt to reduce carriage might be ill advised. Recently, studies have shown that microbiota diversity and certain members of the Clostridia class, such as *Lachnospiraceae* and *Ruminococcaceae*, are consistently associated with gastrointestinal health.[8,10,18] Maintaining diversity and increasing the abundance of these Clostridia could be a potential target of probiotic development. In horses, to date only one study has assessed the effect of probiotics on the composition of the microbiota in a small number of foals. A significant effect was not seen.[19]

REGULATION OF COMMERCIAL PROBIOTICS AND QUALITY CONTROL

In North America (NA), most commercial probiotics are sold over the counter, without published efficacy or safety studies or ongoing quality control. In the United States, probiotics, also called *direct-fed microbials*, can be classified as a drug or as a dietary or feed supplement. If classified as a drug, the product needs to be approved and undergo quality control based on rules set forth by the Food and Drug Administration (FDA). Currently there are no approved probiotic products classified as drugs for horses in NA. If probiotics are classified as dietary or feed supplement, they fall under the category, "generally regarded as safe (GRAS)," and do not need to go through FDA drug-level approval. The FDA requires that supplements be labeled in a truthful and not misleading manner. The producers just provide an expert opinion on why the product should be considered GRAS and be approved by the FDA. The labels need to contain information to identify the feed additive, its concentration, and details on its safe and effective use. Claims that a feed additive can be used to cure, treat, or prevent disease named expressed or implied care are not allowed. The Center for Veterinary Medicine of the FDA, however, permits the use of meaningful health information; for example, "gastrointestinal health" claims on horse feed fall under this policy. Consequently, in NA, there are numerous probiotic products for use in horses on the market that can be obtained over the counter and claim to benefit the horse in various ways. Peer-reviewed published studies proving the efficacy of these products, however, are limited or in most cases lacking.

Even though the FDA regulates the labeling of probiotic products, many commercial veterinary and human probiotic preparations are not accurately represented by label claims. Studies evaluating labels of detailed contents of human and veterinary products showed that only 43% of human products and 8% of veterinary products from Canada were adequately labeled. There were inadequate descriptions of the bacterial content, including missing names, unspecified strains, nonexisting names, potentially pathogenic genera (eg, *Staphylococcus*) and outdated names.[20,21] Quality control of the active ingredient of commercial probiotics is also poor. Only 15% of veterinary and human probiotics contained the specified organism at the label claimed concentrations. Some products were missing organisms entirely or contained too little or too much of an active ingredient (0%–215% of the claimed amounts). All veterinary products contained less than 2% of the listed concentration of bacteria.[22] The effect of probiotics in a clinical setting might, therefore, not be predictable due to inadequate and inconsistent content of commercial probiotic formulations. Currently available published or claimed results of studies are likely also affected by this poor quality control. Commercial products used in research studies and evaluated as part of such, contained up to 100 times less active ingredient than what was claimed on the label.[23] The lack of effect seen in this particular study could be due to the inadequate content of the product rather than actual lack of biological effect. Even when using specifically designed (self-made) formulations, the content can be inadequate due to storage or production issues, and should be evaluated.[19]

MECHANISMS OF ACTION OF PROBIOTICS

Proposed mechanisms for the effect of probiotics include modulation of the host immune system, production of antimicrobial substances, inhibition or inactivation of bacterial toxins, displacement of pathogenic microorganisms (competitive exclusion), improvement in micronutrient absorption, and improvement in epithelial barrier function (**Fig. 1**).

The local intestinal and general immune system, including innate and adaptive responses are influenced by probiotics.[24] Conserved recognition receptors of the intestinal epithelial cells (IECs) and gut-associated immune cells recognize probiotics, and their metabolites, process them and evoke a signaling cascade. The effects include maintenance and fortification of the intestinal barrier by maintaining tight junctions, production of mucus, and survival and growth of IECs. This results in a stronger mucosal barrier against invading pathogens. Furthermore, the gut associated lymphoid follicles are presented with components of the probiotic strains by antigen presenting cells and induce differentiating of B cells into plasma cells. As a result, IgA, which is important for mucosal immunity, is released into the intestinal lumen

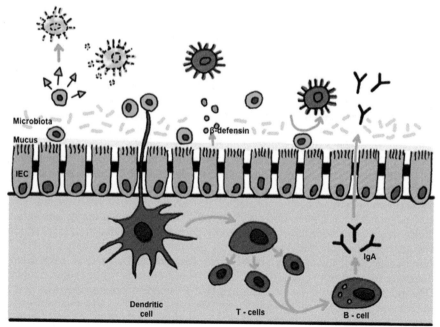

Fig. 1. Mechanism of action of probiotics. Green, probiotic; purple, pathogen.

by plasma cells.[25] The IgA and β-defensin, produced and released by IECs results in suppression of growth of pathogens as well as systemic and local anti-inflammatory effects.[24] Probiotics also modify the cytokine production by IECs and cells of the innate immune system, such as macrophages and dendritic cells, and therefore show an anti-inflammatory effect.[26] Systemically, probiotics can influence immuno-globulin production by altering systemic immunoglobulin isotope profiles.[27] Most of these studies assessing the effects of probiotics on the host have been conducted using human or laboratory animal cell lines, but to date no similar studies for horses have been published. Given the close conservation of the immune system across species, it is likely that similar effects do occur in horses.

Some probiotic strains produce antimicrobial metabolites in large quantities. These include fatty acids, lactic acid, and acetic acid. Other antimicrobial substances, such as formic acids, free fatty acids, ammonia, hydrogen peroxide, diacetyl, bacteriolytic enzymes, bacteriocins, antibiotics, and several undefined substances, are produced in much smaller amounts.[28]

Competitive exclusion refers to the ability of probiotic strains to decrease the amount of pathogens present in the intestinal lumen and their capacity to adhere to epithelial cells. Probiotic strains adhere to epithelial cells, block receptors and increase mucin production. Subsequently pathogens can no longer adhere or gain entrance into epithelial cells.[29] Additionally, probiotic strains occupy ecological niches and compete for nutrients, thus making it more difficult for pathogenic bacteria to survive in the gastrointestinal lumen.

Toxins are important and well-described virulence factors for enteropathogenic bacteria. Probiotics have been shown to inactivate toxins, reduce toxin production, and sometimes render toxigenic enteropathogens nonpathogenic.[30] The antitoxin effect of some probiotics may be beneficial in positively managing infectious diarrhea.

SAFETY OF PROBIOTICS

Adverse effects of probiotic administration have been rarely reported. In humans, the few reports available describe extraintestinal infections rather than enteric disease.[31]

Fungaemia due to treatment with S boulardii has been reported in human neo-nates.[32] Whether this could be a problem in horses is unknown, because studies with S boulardii in equine neonates have not been performed.[33]

Probiotics typically are used in individuals with enteric disease and adverse enteric consequences might be hard to distinguish from the primary disease present. It is reasonable to assume that the incidence of adverse events is very low, consistent with the GRAS classification of probiotics. In adult horses, there are no published reports of enteric disease after probiotic administration.[12,34] Doses are generally extrapolated from human recommendations and adjusted by weight.[13,35] Even administration of up to three times the manufacturers' recommended doses to healthy horses did not result in any adverse effects.[36] The effect of probiotics in horses with enteric disease might differ from the effect in healthy horses, but no adverse clinical effects have so far been reported in horses with gastrointestinal diseases either.[13,33,36] Most investigators, therefore, consider probiotics safe to be used in healthy and diseased adult horses.

The safety of probiotic use in foals has to be assessed independently of adults because there are major differences in immune system function and gastrointestinal microbiota composition between adults and foals.[37] Particularly, during the first month, the diversity is significantly decreased compared with older foals.[38] Although several published studies demonstrate safety of commercially available and self-made probiotics in foals,[34,39] there are also reports on adverse enteric effects.[19,35] In both cited studies a self-made probiotic was evaluated as a preventative measure for neonatal diarrhea in a placebo-controlled trial. The treatment group showed increased incidence of diarrhea and need for veterinary intervention in both studies.[35,40] Although it is unclear why these foals developed diarrhea, the immature microbiota of the foals could have allowed overgrowth of lactic acid bacteria, resulting in osmotic imbalances and diarrhea. Alternatively, the probiotics could have changed the microbiota to allow for pathogen adhesion to epithelial cells. The microbiota remains relatively stable in foals after two months of life but compared with adult horses differences are still present[38]; therefore, probiotic administration to foals more than two months old is less likely to result in severe side effects. Probiotics should be used with caution in foals, and safety studies should be performed before a product is administered.

CURRENT EVIDENCE FOR PROBIOTIC EFFICACY IN TREATMENT OR PREVENTION OF EQUINE GASTROINTESTINAL DISEASE

Probiotics have been administered to adult horses with acute enteropathies and to decrease Salmonella shedding. Although some studies have shown beneficial effects of probiotics, other studies could not corroborate these results (**Fig. 2**).[13,23,33,36,41–43] Overall, few studies are available, and these cannot be compared easily due to differences in study design, outcome parameters, and formulations used. Often one outcome parameter was influenced positively, such as duration of diarrhea; however, no effect on mortality or duration of hospitalization was seen. The more outcome parameters studied, the more likely significant effects are observed. Consequently, to date, the overall evidence is weak. The effect of a probiotic in a specific clinical context is likely unique to that context. The effect of a probiotic in horses with a specific disease cannot be extrapolated from results of studies in healthy horses or on horses with another disease. Also, extrapolation from humans or other species should not be done. Because clinical context is important, studies on the use of probiotics should ideally define the study population (healthy horses, horses with a specific disease, and so forth) and fully describe the probiotic (exact strain, dose, dosage regimen, and manufacturing details).

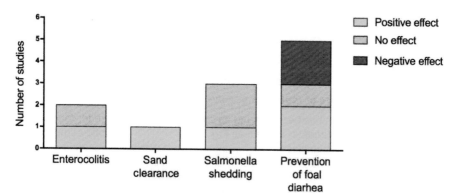

Fig. 2. Summary of effects of probiotics on preventing or treating gastrointestinal disease in horses.

Use of Probiotics for Treatment of Acute Enterocolitis in Adult Horses

S boulardii has been used with equivocal results. In one randomized, blinded, placebo-controlled clinical trial, horses receiving the probiotic had a shorter duration of diarrhea and watery diarrhea but not loose feces.[13] Despite this potential positive effect, the results of this study must be interpreted with caution, because there was no difference between the groups in relation to outcome, duration of hospitalization, and recurrence of diarrhea. In addition to the confounding factor of additional treatments, the number of cases was low, with only seven horses in each group.[13] In the second randomized placebo-controlled clinical trial involving 12 horses, no significant differences were observed between groups for occurrence of normal fecal consistency or cessation of watery diarrhea.[33] Also, days to improvement in attitude, resolution of leukopenia, appetite, normalization of heart rate, respiratory rate, and temperature, length of stay in hospital, survival to discharge, and occurrence of secondary complications were not different between groups.[33] Although this study was influenced by fewer confounding factors and evaluated more clinical variables compared with the previously cited study,[13] the number of cases was low and adjunct treatment was variable among horses, making interpretation of the results more difficult. Although both studies investigated the same probiotic, they are difficult to compare due to a heterogeneous horse population and different inclusion and outcome criteria. In summary, the evidence for an effect of S boulardii as an adjunctive treatment of enterocolitis in horses is weak. Additional probiotic strains have not been studied in adult horses with acute enterocolitis. Overall studies in horses provided weak evidence for the use of probiotics.

Salmonella Infection and Shedding

In horses, the effect of probiotics on Salmonella shedding has been investigated but results have been disappointing to date. No differences in Salmonella shedding rates, prevalence of postoperative diarrhea, leukopenia, length of antimicrobial therapy, and length of hospitalization were found between groups.[36,41] The overall number of horses shedding Salmonella was small, fecal samples were taken at irregular, arbitrary intervals, and, given that Salmonella shedding can be intermittent, some cases might have been missed.[23,44] These limitations could have influenced the results of these study. In contrast, administration of a probiotic decreased the incidence of Salmonella shedding by 65% in another study, but the difference was not significant ($P = .19$) due to low power of the study.[23] In other species, it is known that the effect of probiotics depends on the agent studied, and so far few probiotics have been evaluated in horses. Additional studies are necessary before excluding the beneficial effects of probiotics on Salmonella shedding in horses. There is currently little evidence supporting the use of probiotics to decrease Salmonella shedding or salmonellosis in horses.

Current Evidence for use of Probiotics in Foals

Probiotic administration has been studied as a preventative measure for foal diarrhea in several studies with variable results (see **Fig. 2**).[35,39,40,45,46] Probiotic administration was associated with a significantly higher incidence of diarrhea, presence of clinical signs (lethargy, fever, and anorexia colic) and the need for veterinary examination and treatment in two studies.[35,40] In another study, foals in the probiotic group showed statistically significant larger weight gain after treatment and a significantly lower incidence of diarrhea.[39] These effects, however, were only significant at specific time points. It is unlikely that the diarrhea was clinically important as evidenced by a lack of difference in the need for medical intervention between the 2 groups. In a fourth study on prevention of neonatal diarrhea in foals, a reduction of diarrhea incidence by 60% could be achieved with probiotic administration.[45] Although this result seems promising, there were several limitations to this study, including unequal treatment groups and inconsistent monitoring (every two weeks), which could have resulted in oversight of many diarrhea episodes. Additionally it is unclear how often foals were treated with the probiotic and the study was not blinded. In another study, *Bacillus cereus* supplementation did not have an effect on incidence of diarrhea during the first 58 days of life in a study in 25 foals, irrespective of the dose used.[46] These studies cannot be directly compared because different products were used. In summary, every probiotic product that is used in neonatal foals should be evaluated for safety and efficacy before administration. Larger-scale controlled studies of different strains and products are necessary before conclusions can be drawn on the clinical efficacy of probiotics in foals with diarrhea.

FECAL MICROBIAL TRANSPLANTATION

All current probiotics consist of one or a few strains that comprise a minor component of the intestinal microbiota. Therefore, they might have limited ability to influence the entire gastrointestinal microbiota. Scientists and clinicians are now evaluating the other end of the probiotic complexity spectrum, fecal transplants. Fecal transplants consist of an intact, highly complex microbial community composed by thousands of species. Fecal microbial transplantation constitutes the transfer a fecal suspension from a healthy donor into the bowel of the recipient. Fecal microbial transplantation has been shown to be highly effective in treating recurrent *Clostridium difficile* infections in humans. Although there are no published studies or abstracts in horses, anecdotal reports suggest that this form of therapy also might be effective in horses with acute colitis or chronic diarrhea.[47,48]

SUMMARY

Although probiotics have shown promise in treatment of selected diseases in humans, the evidence in horses is weak. For any given disease, only few probiotic organisms have been evaluated so far and most studies were underpowered or confounded. On the basis of examination of existing data, no specific product can be recommended for use. The aim of developing the one probiotic to aid in prevention or treatment of all diseases is unrealistic. The choice and combination of strains for a therapeutic formulation needs to be specific for each disease and should be based on the in vitro properties of the strains and tested in clinical placebo controlled randomized trials. Based on lack of regulation regarding quality control of commercial products, use of over-the-counter products is questionable, particularly in the absence of scientific information on safety and clinical efficacy. Probiotics likely have a different effect in foals because the gastrointestinal microbiota transitions to the adult microbiota during the first months of life. Adverse effects have been reported in foals and probiotics should be evaluated for safety before use in foals. Despite all these limitations, probiotics generally are regarded as safe, and easy to administer. Therefore, additional research is warranted to test possible applications in equine veterinary practice. Exploiting new knowledge of the composition of the equine microbiota, the focus of probiotic research should shift from currently used agents to species that are abundant in the intestinal microbiota of the horse. By combining microbiota research, research on fecal microbial transplantation and probiotic research, a designer probiotic containing all beneficial microbes could eventually be developed.

REFERENCES

1. Metchnikoff E. Optimistic studies. New York: Putman's Sons; 1908. p. 22.
2. FAO/WHO. Working group for drafting guidelines for the evaluation of probiotics in food. 2002. Available at: ftp://ftp.fao.org/es/esn/food/wgreport2.pdf. Accessed December 12, 2017.
3. Kailasapathy K, Chin J. Survival and therapeutic potential of probiotic organisms with reference to Lactobacillus acidophilus and Bifidobacterium spp. Immunol Cell Biol 2000;78:80–8.
4. Ogue-Bon E, Khoo C, McCartney AL, et al. In vitro effects of synbiotic fermentation on the canine faecal microbiota. FEMS Microbiol Ecol 2010;73:587–600.
5. Biourge V, Vallet C, Levesque A, et al. The use of probiotics in the diet of dogs. J Nutr 1998;128:2730S–2S.
6. Dougal K, de la Fuente G, Harris PA, et al. Identification of a core bacterial community within the large intestine of the horse. PLoS One 2013;8:e77660.
7. Dougal K, Harris PA, Edwards A, et al. A comparison of the microbiome and the metabolome of different regions of the equine hindgut. FEMS Microbiol Ecol 2012;82:642–52.
8. Costa MC, Arroyo LG, Allen-Vercoe E, et al. Comparison of the fecal microbiota of healthy horses and horses with colitis by high throughput sequencing of the V3-V5 region of the 16S rRNA gene. PLoS One 2012;7:e41484.
9. Minamoto Y, Otoni CC, Steelman SM, et al. Alteration of the fecal microbiota and serum metabolite profiles in dogs with idiopathic inflammatory bowel disease. Gut Microbes 2015;6:33–47.
10. Suchodolski JS. Diagnosis and interpretation of intestinal dysbiosis in dogs and cats. Vet J 2016;215:30–7.
11. Weese JS, Holcombe SJ, Embertson RM, et al. Changes in the faecal microbiota of mares precede the development of postpartum colic. Equine Vet J 2014;47: 641–9.
12. Weese JS, Anderson ME, Lowe A, et al. Preliminary investigation of the probiotic potential of Lactobacillus rhamnosus strain GG in horses: fecal recovery following oral administration and safety. Can Vet J 2003;44:299–302.
13. Desrochers AM, Dolente BA, Roy MF, et al. Efficacy of Saccharomyces boulardii for treatment of horses with acute enterocolitis. J Am Vet Med Assoc 2005;227: 954–9.
14. Medina B, Girard ID, Jacotot E, et al. Effect of a preparation of Saccharomyces cerevisiae on microbial profiles and fermentation patterns in the large intestine of horses fed a high fiber or a high starch diet. J Anim Sci 2002;80:2600–9.
15. Jouany JP, Gobert J, Medina B, et al. Effect of live yeast culture supplementation on apparent digestibility and rate of passage in horses fed a high-fiber or high-starch diet. J Anim Sci 2008;86:339–47.
16. Jouany JP, Medina B, Bertin G, et al. Effect of live yeast culture supplementation on hindgut microbial communities and their polysaccharidase and glycoside hydrolase activities in horses fed a high-fiber or high-starch diet. J Anim Sci 2009; 87:2844–52.
17. Schoster A, Staempfli HR, Arroyo LG, et al. Longitudinal study of Clostridium difficile and antimicrobial susceptibility of Escherichia coli in healthy horses in a community setting. Vet Microbiol 2012;159:364–70.
18. Schoster A, Mosing M, Jalali M, et al. Effects of transport, fasting and anaesthesia on the faecal microbiota of healthy adult horses. Equine Vet J 2016;48:595–602.

19. Schoster A, Guardabassi L, Staempfli HR, et al. The longitudinal effect of a multi-strain probiotic on the intestinal bacterial microbiota of neonatal foals. Equine Vet J 2016;6:689–96.
20. Weese JS, Martin H. Assessment of commercial probiotic bacterial contents and label accuracy. Can Vet J 2011;52:43–6.
21. Weese JS. Evaluation of deficiencies in labeling of commercial probiotics. Can Vet J 2003;44:982–3.
22. Weese JS. Microbiologic evaluation of commercial probiotics. J Am Vet Med Assoc 2002;220:794–7.
23. Ward MP, Alinovi CA, Couetil LL, et al. A Randomized clinical trial using probiotics to prevent Salmonella fecal shedding in hospitalized horses. J Equine Vet Sci 2004;24:242–7.
24. Oelschlaeger TA. Mechanisms of probiotic actions - A review. Int J Med Microbiol 2010;300:57–62.
25. Park JH, Um JI, Lee BJ, et al. Encapsulated Bifidobacterium bifidum potentiates intestinal IgA production. Cell Immunol 2002;219:22–7.
26. Watanabe T, Nishio H, Tanigawa T, et al. Probiotic Lactobacillus casei strain Shirota prevents indomethacin-induced small intestinal injury: involvement of lactic acid. Am J Physiol Gastrointest Liver Physiol 2009;297:G506–13.
27. Thomas CM, Versalovic J. Probiotics-host communication: modulation of signaling pathways in the intestine. Gut Microbes 2010;1:148–63.
28. Saarela M, Mogensen G, Fonden R, et al. Probiotic bacteria: safety, functional and technological properties. J Biotechnol 2000;84:197–215.
29. Collado MC, Grzeskowiak L, Salminen S. Probiotic strains and their combination inhibit in vitro adhesion of pathogens to pig intestinal mucosa. Curr Microbiol 2007;55:260–5.
30. Chen X, Kokkotou EG, Mustafa N, et al. Saccharomyces boulardii inhibits ERK1/2 mitogen-activated protein kinase activation both in vitro and in vivo and protects against Clostridium difficile toxin A-induced enteritis. J Biol Chem 2006;281:24449–54.
31. Shanahan F. A commentary on the safety of probiotics. Gastroenterol Clin North Am 2012;41:869–76.
32. Chioukh FZ, Ben Hmida H, Ben Ameur K, et al. Saccharomyces cerevisiae fungemia in a premature neonate treated receiving probiotics. Med Mal Infect 2013;43(8):359–60 [in French].
33. Boyle AG, Magdesian KG, Durando MM, et al. Saccharomyces boulardii viability and efficacy in horses with antimicrobial-induced diarrhoea. Vet Rec 2013;172:128.
34. Weese JS, Anderson ME, Lowe A, et al. Screening of the equine intestinal microflora for potential probiotic organisms. Equine Vet J 2004;36:351–5.
35. Weese JS, Rousseau J. Evaluation of Lactobacillus pentosus WE7 for prevention of diarrhea in neonatal foals. J Am Vet Med Assoc 2005;226:2031–4.
36. Parraga ME, Spier SJ, Thurmond M, et al. A clinical trial of probiotic administration for prevention of Salmonella shedding in the postoperative period in horses with colic. J Vet Intern Med 1997;11:36–41.
37. Earing JE. Bacterial colonization of the equine gut; comparison of mare and foal Pairs by PCR-DGGE. Adv Microbiol 2012;02:79–86.
38. Costa MC, Stampfli HR, Allen-Vercoe E, et al. Development of the faecal microbiota in foals. Equine Vet J 2016;48:681–8.
39. Yuyama T. Evaluation of a host-specific Lactobacillus probiotic in neonatal foals. Intern J Appl Res Vet Med 2004;2:26–33.

40. Schoster A, Staempfli HR, Abrahams M, et al. Effect of a probiotic on prevention of diarrhea and clostridium difficile and clostridium perfringens shedding in foals. J Vet Intern Med 2015;29:925–31.
41. Kim LM, Morley PS, Traub-Dargatz JL, et al. Factors associated with Salmonella shedding among equine colic patients at a veterinary teaching hospital. J Am Vet Med Assoc 2001;218:740–8.
42. Landes AD, Hassel DM, Funk JD, et al. Fecal sand clearance is enhanced with a product combining probiotics, prebiotics, and psyllium in clinically normal horses. J Equine Vet Sci 2008;28:79–84.
43. Ishizaka S, Matsuda A, Amagai Y, et al. Oral administration of fermented probiotics improves the condition of feces in adult horses. J Equine Sci 2014;25:65–72.
44. van Duijkeren E, Flemming C, Sloet van Oldruitenborgh-Oosterbaan M, et al. Diagnosing salmonellosis in horses. Culturing of multiple versus single faecal samples. Vet Q 1995;17:63–6.
45. Tanabe S, Suzuki T, Wasano Y, et al. Anti-inflammatory and intestinal barrier-protective activities of commensal lactobacilli and bifidobacteria in thoroughbreds: role of probiotics in diarrhea prevention in neonatal thoroughbreds. J Equine Sci 2014;25:37–43.
46. John J, Roediger K, Schroedl W, et al. Development of intestinal microflora and occurrence of diarrhoea in sucking foals: effects of bacillus cereus var. toyoi supplementation. BMC Vet Res 2015;11:34.
47. Feary DJ, Hassel DM. Enteritis and colitis in horses. Vet Clin North Am Equine Pract 2006;22:437–79.
48. Mullen K, Yasuda K, Divers JT, et al. Equine faecal microbiota transplant: current knowledge, proposed guidelines, and future directions. Equine Vet Edu 2016. [Epub ahead of print].

Techniques and Accuracy of Abdominal Ultrasound in Gastrointestinal Diseases of Horses and Foals

Nicola C. Cribb, MA, VetMB, DVSc,
Luis G. Arroyo, Lic. Med. Vet, DVSc, PhD*

KEYWORDS

- Equine • Gastrointestinal disease • Colic • Ultrasonography • Accuracy • Sensitivity
- Specificity

KEY POINTS

- Abdominal ultrasound is a useful aid in the diagnosis of equine gastrointestinal disease.
- Sensitivity, specificity, and positive and negative predictive values of ultrasonography in the diagnosis of disease are necessary to determine the accuracy of this imaging modality.
- Techniques to identify various components of the gastrointestinal tract are well described in horses.

TECHNIQUES

Introduction

A thorough examination of the gastrointestinal (GI) tract in horses relies on clinical examination, ancillary diagnostic tests and procedures such as per rectal examination, peritoneal fluid analysis and diagnostic imaging. Since the inaugural research publication on the use of ultrasound (US) in the diagnostic evaluation of patients with colic in 1997,[1] a wealth of literature has developed describing techniques for identifying GI disease in horses and foals. Ultrasonography has become one of the most-used diagnostic imaging modalities under referral and field conditions. The design and development of light, portable machines with powerful software and high-quality images have turned this piece of equipment into an attractive and profitable investment for field service practitioners and referral centers. The techniques used to examine and assess the different intra-abdominal organs and viscera in adult horses and foals have been thoroughly described in textbooks and research articles.[2–4] Therefore, only a

Department of Clinical Studies, Ontario Veterinary College, University of Guelph, 50 Stone Road East, Guelph, Ontario N1G 2W1, Canada
* Corresponding author.
E-mail address: larroyo@uoguelph.ca

Vet Clin Equine 34 (2018) 25–38
https://doi.org/10.1016/j.cveq.2017.11.001
0749-0739/18/© 2017 Elsevier Inc. All rights reserved.

vetequine.theclinics.com

brief description for routine scanning and anatomic landmarks is included. The main focus of this article is on the accuracy and usefulness of this imaging modality to assist with the diagnosis of GI disorders in foals and adult horses.

Patient Preparation

A thorough or partial abdominal examination of the abdomen of standing or recumbent adult horses and foals can be performed. Horses should ideally be secured in stocks where they can be safely scanned. Portable US machines have made it possible to scan horses while standing in the stall, hallway, or even while walking, which can be useful for horses displaying overt signs of colic.

A common practice is to soak the hair and skin with 70% isopropyl ethanol in order to facilitate coupling between the probe and the skin. In horses with thick and long-hair coats (ie, during winter months in the northern hemisphere), it may be difficult to obtain good-quality images. Areas of particular interest are better visualized by clipping the hair over the targeted structure. There are several factors that could affect how patients are examined, which largely depend on how cooperative the patients are, the degree of pain, and the differential diagnoses considered. A thorough examination is usually recommended to collect as much information of the entire GI tract as possible; however, in some cases only a partial examination can be performed. A protocol for fast localized abdominal sonography (FLASH system) for horses admitted with colic was developed and is considered useful in detecting major intra-abdominal abnormalities even by inexperienced operators.[5] It is useful in some cases to perform multiple US examinations. The repeatability of identifying a particular abdominal structure on selected locations performed in multiple horses in repeated examinations has been assessed.[6] Some segments of the GI tract, such as the caecum and sacculated large intestine (LI), can be more consistently identified during abdominal examinations than other segments. In some animals, the sacculated colon is occasionally identified in dorsal flank sites; the location of the small intestine (SI) can be both variable and require repeated examinations.[6]

Principles of Disease that can be Used for Examination of the Gastrointestinal Tract by Ultrasonography

There are several physical abnormal changes that can be used to enhance information obtained by US evaluation. These changes include displacements of the normal topographic anatomic arrangements of the GI tract and changes in motility (peristalsis), bowel wall thickness, layering, contents, shape, and diameter.

Anatomic abnormalities

The equine LI has several anatomic features that lend itself to diagnostic ultrasonography use. In brief, the large colon is composed of 4 segments, the right and left ventral colons and the right and left dorsal colons, with the only mesenteric attachment to the body wall being between the aboral portion of the right dorsal colon and the dorsal body wall. The large colon can, therefore, move into different abnormal positions throughout the abdomen causing vascular compromises, distensions, and outflow obstructions. The ventral colon is sacculated, whereas the dorsal colon is nonsacculated; this can be exploited for the identification of colon positioning.[7] The blood supply to the large colon travels along the medial aspect of the colon in the mesocolon. Similarly, the identification of colonic vasculature in an abnormal lateral position can suggest abnormal colon positioning.[8] Knowledge of normal positioning of the cecum and colon can also help differentiate between different types of intussusceptions affecting these parts of the LI.[9]

Alterations in bowel thickness

The nature of disease of some conditions of the large colon also allow for identification by US examination. For example, thickening of the colonic wall from vascular leakage as a result of the venous outflow obstruction during a strangulating volvulus of the large colon can be identified.[10]

The normal range in wall thickness throughout all segments of the GI tract in horses is well described, and reference ranges have been established. It is usually the increase, not decrease, in thickness of a particular segment of the GI tract that the clinician is assessing while scanning (**Fig. 1**A). Bowel thickness can be increased as a result of intramural accumulation of fluids and protein transudate from occluded or damaged microvasculature such as in a large colon volvulus or enterocolitis. Inflammatory processes, such as in colitis, around encysted cyathostomins, and infiltrative bowel disease, can cause wall thickening (**Fig. 2**A). *Lawsonia intracellularis* and idiopathic muscular hypertrophy SI proliferative disorders often result in thickening of segments of the SI of various lengths (**Fig. 2**B). Some neoplastic disorders can cause focal or diffuse infiltration of the GI tract, such as squamous cell carcinomas in the stomach and enteric lymphoma involving the SI, which can be visualized by US and aid on the diagnostic workup of these conditions.

Other ultrasonography abnormalities, such as bowel wall thinning and intramural gas, have been reported in people.[11] Intramural gas has been reported in foals as well, but no other confirmatory tests for the ultrasonographic images were reported.[4]

Alterations in intestinal motility

Rhythmic peristaltic movements can be seen during real-time US examination, and the range of contractions for normal horses has been recorded.[2] The lack of or incomplete contractions of the intestine are commonly used to aid in the diagnosis of complete or partial obstructions (ie, SI volvulus) and functional disorders (Duodenitis-Proximal Jejunitis [DPJ], grass sickness). Increased motility can also be assessed and are commonly observed in horses with enterocolitis for example.

Distension

Distended bowel often occurs oral to the site of an obstruction.[2] Distended SI is often seen in the ventral portion of the abdomen where it comes to lay from being weighed down by fluid accumulations within its lumen (**Fig. 1**B).

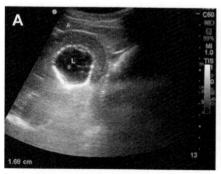 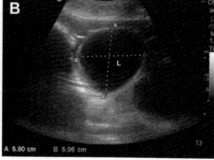

Fig. 1. Ultrasonographic images from a 9-year-old warmblood mare evaluated with signs of acute colic. (*A*) Markedly thickened SI segment (wall thickness 1.68 cm) due to congestion and edema caused by a strangulating lipoma are shown. (*B*) Markedly distended SI segment presumed oral to the strangulated portion of the intestine. Both images were obtained with a SonoSite, C60×/2- to 5-MHz convex transducer (Fujifilm SonoSite, Inc, Bothell, Washington) on the cranio-ventral side of the abdomen. L, lumen.

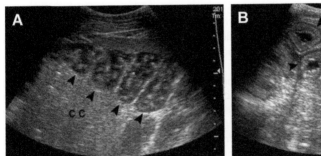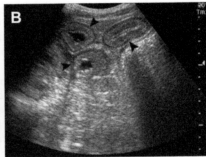

Fig. 2. Sonograms from a 1-year-old Thoroughbred filly evaluated because of severe hypoproteinemia and diarrhea. (*A*) Markedly thickened colonic wall due to inflammation and edema caused by a massive number of encysted cyathostomins. Black arrowheads denote edematous colonic folds protruding into the lumen. (*B*) Markedly thickened SI segments (*black arrowheads*) due to *Lawsonia intracellularis* infection (proliferative enteropathy). The upper portion of the image represents the abdominal wall. Both images were obtained with an ATL HDI 5000 (Philips Medical Systems, Markham, Ontario) C5-2 MHz convex transducer on the midventral lateral right side of the abdomen. C, colon contents.

Equipment for Ultrasound Examination of the Gastrointestinal Tract

Adult horses and foals can be scanned with variable-frequency US probes with (2–5 MHz); however, linear or convex high-frequency (5.0–7.5 MHz) probes can be used in foals.

Topographic Anatomic Locations for Identifying Abnormalities of the Following Sections of the Gastrointestinal Tract

Stomach

The stomach can be found dorsal to the spleen and ventral to the lung in the left 10th to 15th intercostal spaces (ICS). Imaging of the stomach wall is limited to part of the greater curvature, which appears as a large thin semicircular curvilinear line immediately adjacent and medial to the spleen. In equine neonates, the stomach can be visualized between the 6th and 12th ICS approximately midway between the dorsum and the ventrum and more ventral in the cranial abdomen. The liquid contents can be visualized during the first days of life; but soon, within a week, the ingesta are no more visible, similar to adults.[12]

Duodenum

The duodenum is usually easily identified because of its attachments and close proximity to other organs. It travels between the liver and the right dorsal colon toward the caudal aspect of the right kidney where it crosses toward the left side of the abdomen. This segment of the duodenum is consistently imaged between the 14th and 17th intercostal spaces along its trajectory slightly dorsal to an imaginary line between the olecranon and the tuber sacrale.[13] The caudal lung field can interfere while scanning as it moves back and forth into the scanning field.

Jejunum

The jejunum can be consistently found dorsal to the left dorsal colon and in one or more ventral locations. It can be also found, but not consistently, on the left and right ventral caudal regions, the right ventral cranial and flank regions, the right and left ventral middle regions, the left ventral cranial and gastrosplenic regions, and the caudo-dorsal to the spleen region.[14] In general, its highly variable in how frequently and where the SI (jejunum or ileum) is identified; but the ventral sites are most consistent.[6]

Ileum

The ileum can be inconsistently imaged in the ventral abdomen in adult horses because of its anatomic location in the medial and cranial aspect of the cecum.

Cecum and Large Colon

The cecum is visualized in the right caud-odorsal quadrant (paralumbar fossa) and can be followed to its apex toward the ventral abdomen. This LI segment is recognized for its semicurved and sacculated appearance with an approximately 3-mm wall thickness. The right dorsal colon has a nonsacculated appearance, and the normal wall thickness is less than 3.5 mm^2; but there is a wide range of variability on the wall thickness along the different intercostal spaces. The presence of gas in the lumen prevents imaging of the contents except in some conditions, such as typhlitis/colitis. Inexperienced operators can mistake a fluid-filled large colon for SI in neonates.

Small colon

It is possible to visualize the small colon in the left caudo-dorsal quadrant by transabdominal US; however, it can be more easily imaged transrectally. It has sacculations and, therefore, a similar ultrasonographic appearance to the LI. The diameter ranges between 7 and 10 cm, and the contents can also vary in consistency.[15]

Rectum

Transrectal US can be used to examine some intra-abdominal structures/organs, including parts of the GI tract, such as the small colon, cecum, and parts of the large colon (ie, pelvic flexure). Rectal US had been used to aid in the diagnosis and provide follow-up information on perirectal abscesses[16,17]

ASSESSMENT OF ACCURACY OF ABDOMINAL ULTRASOUND IN DIAGNOSING DISEASES IN THE GASTROINTESTINAL TRACT OF HORSES

A search of the PubMed database for reports of horses and foals with GI disease, that used ultrasonography as part of a diagnostic process, reveals at least 51 publications, including case reports, case series, and retrospective as well as prospective studies. A rigorous evaluation process of diagnostic tests before acceptance into clinical practice is necessary to avoid incorrect treatment decisions,[18] and this is in part achieved by a critical assessment of accuracy. The accuracy of a diagnostic test is the degree to which it actually represents what it is intended to represent.[19]

Reference Standard

In studies of diagnostic accuracy, the outcome from the test under evaluation is compared with the outcome of the reference standard, also known as gold standard. The reference standard is considered to be the best available method for establishing the presence or absence of the condition of interest; in the horse with GI disease, this is often colic surgery or necropsy. In some instances, a concrete gold standard is not available, such as a colic that has resolved with medical therapy; other approaches must be relied on to assess accuracy. As an example, ultrasonography as a test for detecting sand accumulations in horses was compared with radiography as the reference standard.[20] An evaluation of the validity of the reference standard measurement must be made to assess how well the measurement represents the disease of interest. For the aforementioned study, radiography has previously been shown to be efficacious in detecting sand accumulations.[21] However, in a different study, histology of rectal biopsy as a reference standard was used to assess ultrasonographically measured SI wall thickness as a test for inflammatory bowel disease.[22] The disease may not have been truly represented by this choice of reference standard, calling into question the usefulness of the assessment of ultrasonography as a diagnostic tool.[23] In the necessity to use a valid reference standard, many reports include only horses that were examined at surgery or necropsy; the results and interpretations are then skewed to a more severe presentation of horses with GI disease, so the need for a valid reference standard that may not be the gold standard is real.

Assessing Accuracy

For measurements on a continuous scale, such as thickness of SI, accuracy can be determined from the mean difference between the measurement under investigation and the reference standard across study subjects.[19] For measurements on a categorical scale, such as mild, moderate, and severe degrees of thickness of the intestinal wall, accuracy can be determined from the specificity and sensitivity of the measurement with respect to the reference standard, which is usually findings at the celiotomy or necropsy examination.

Sensitivity is defined as the proportion of horses with the disease in which the test gives the correct answer (it is positive).

$$Sensitivity = \frac{number\ of\ test\ positive}{Number\ of\ reference\ standard\ positive}$$

The specificity is the proportion of horses without the disease in which the test gives the correct answer (it is negative).

$$Specficity = \frac{number\ of\ test\ negatives}{Number\ of\ reference\ standard\ negatives}$$

This can be determined by a simple 2 × 2 table (**Table 1**). Sensitivity and specificity can, therefore, be used to quantify the diagnostic ability of the test. However, in clinical practice the test result is all that is known,[22] so it is useful to know how good the test is at predicting abnormality; predictive values provide information on this.

The positive predictive value (PPV) is the proportion of patients with positive test results who are correctly diagnosed as being positive. The negative predictive value (NPV) is the proportion of patients with negative test results who are correctly diagnosed as being negative.[24]

Table 1
A simple 2 × 2 table with hypothetical sample sizes demonstrating calculation of sensitivity, specifically, positive value, and negative predictive value

US test result		Reference Standard			
		Disease (+)	Disease (−)	Total	
	+	400	60	460	PPV 400/460 = 0.86
	−	40	100	140	NPV 100/140 = 0.72
	Total	440	160	600	—
		Sensitivity 400/440 = 0.9	Specificity 100/160 = 0.62	—	—

Abbreviations: NPV, negative predictive value; PPV, positive predictive value.

Thus, put into a clinical context, the example of assessing how good the US FLASH technique is for diagnosing SI obstruction can be used. When using this technique, is estimated that 80% of horses with SI disease will have dilated, turgid, SI loops (positive result, sensitivity) on US examination, whereas 96% of those without SI obstruction will not have dilated, turgid, SI loops (negative result, specificity) on US examination.[5] Sensitivity and specificity are proportions, and so confidence intervals (CIs) are calculated for them.[22]

The PPV of the same study tells us that 89% of the horses with dilated turgid SI loops had SI obstruction; the NPV tells us that 93% of the horses without dilated turgid SI loops did not have SI obstruction.[5]

The PPV in practice, however, also depends on the prevalence of the abnormality, or type of colic, in the horse being tested. This idea can be appreciated from **Table 1**. This result may vary between different geographic regions or types of clinical practice and may differ from the prevalence in the published study assessing the usefulness of the test.[24]

To further summarize the usefulness of a test, likelihood ratios, diagnostic odds ratios, and the area under a receiver operator curve can be expressed.[19]

Several studies yielding sensitivity, specificity, PPV, and NPV have been reported on for the use of equine diagnostic US for GI diseases in horses. These studies are reviewed in the section on clinical accuracy studies.

Only a few articles report actual numbers of positive/negative test results, reference standards, and also CIs.[10,25,26] A lack of reporting hampers the review and assessment of the study, particularly in instances whereby the results of calculations of sensitivity and specificity cannot be recreated from the reported data. This lack may be due to certain cases being excluded because of low numbers; however, in the authors' opinion this should be clearly stated. Poor reporting has been addressed in the medical literature elsewhere.[18]

Strategies for Enhancing Accuracy

When assessing accuracy, there are 3 main types of measurement error, namely, observer (ultrasonographer) bias, instrument (US machine) bias, and subject (horse) bias.[19] Several strategies can counteract these biases to enhance the accuracy of a diagnostic US test.[19] These strategies include standardization of measurement methods; blinding the ultrasonographer to potential bias from other measurements, such as results of rectal evaluation; training of ultrasonographers; and using appropriate, calibrated US machines. The accuracy studies reviewed in this article manage observer bias by measuring intraobserver and interobserver variability.[10,26]

Further limitations exist in developing assessments of the accuracy of US examination by the nature of clinical cases. These limitations include a lack of control of the timing between the diagnostic US and the reference standard and the treatments administered in between. An example is described in which mesenteric colonic vessels were visualized in a horse that had a 360° large colon torsion.[8] In theory, a 360° torsion should result in normally medially located colonic vessels traveling one full rotation and resuming their original orientation. It is suggested by the investigators of the study, that in this case, the degree of volvulus shifted during the time between sonographic examination and surgery, which is why mesenteric colonic vessels were not visualized with US before surgery.

In general, evaluations of reports of accuracy of diagnostic tests are hampered by lack of key elements of design, conduct, and analysis of studies.[18] Low case numbers, and limitations from the retrospective nature of studies, also prevent statistical analyses of accuracy. The following section is intended to outline the studies that have achieved accuracy assessment in reporting diagnostic methods in equine GI ultrasonography.

CLINICAL ACCURACY STUDIES
How High Should Specificity and Sensitivity Be?

Many accuracy studies report their sensitivity and specificity results as being low, moderate or high. Statistically for this, there is not a defined category, and the value of the test is based on the importance of the result and whether it is more sensitive or more specific than other currently available tests.

Small Intestine Accuracy Studies

Several research groups report on the accuracy of SI ultrasonographic abnormalities for SI disease, as shown in **Table 2**, whether categorized as a lesion, obstruction, or strangulation.

Several associations between ultrasonographic findings and SI disease were described in one study.[28] Not all variables were included in the final model of analysis. Completely distended SI loops, with abnormal motility, thickened SI loops, and increased peritoneal fluid were described as having associations with SI disease, with varied accuracy when analyzed for use as a diagnostic test. Completely distended SI loops had the greatest accuracy.

It seems that absolute lack of motility has the strongest predictive results based on a different study.[1] Other studies describe lower accuracies for this variable based on the presence of false-negative results.[5,28] The high number of false-positive results were in part discussed as reduced SI motility being associated with LI disorders.[28] It is suggested, however, though not based on the outcome of accuracy studies, that SI loops from an SI strangulating obstruction will differ from an LI lesion, as they will be completely distended and with a lack of motility.[28] The term *completely distended* was applied to horses that had a fluid-filled or gas-distended lumen with a round shape as opposed to a square shape.[28]

The presence of thickened distended SI on US was reported as yielding a slightly lower specificity and PPV for SI strangulating obstruction than lack of motility, also due to false-positive results.[1] Included in the study were horses with these signs from peritonitis, intra-abdominal abscessation from previous surgery, or salmonellosis.[1] This finding highlights the necessity of using ultrasonographic findings in conjunction with all other aspects of the clinical examination in determining a diagnosis.

The accuracy of US examination for the identification of SI disease was compared with rectal examination, and it was found that rectal examination was less sensitive than ultrasonography in cases of SI occlusion (51% vs 97%).[27] This type of diagnostic yield study addresses the question of whether a test can be predicted from other information available at the time of the study. A diagnostic yield study can also address the question of whether patients with abnormal results seem to benefit as a direct result of the test being done. To the authors' knowledge, no study has yet looked at this with respect to ultrasonographic techniques in horses with colic.

Large Intestine Accuracy Studies

Left dorsal displacement of the large colon

In a study of 47 horses with left dorsal displacement of the large colon (LDDLC), no controls were included and estimates of diagnostic accuracy were not made.[29] A positive test result in the detection of nephrosplenic entrapment (NSE) was given in each of the following circumstances: dorsal aspect of the spleen obliterated by a gas

Table 2
Specificity and sensitivity, positive predictive value and negative predictive value of ultrasonographically measured variables for different diseases of the equine gastrointestinal tract

Condition	Number of Cases		Measured Variable (n)	SN (%)	SP (%)	PPV (%)	NPV %
	With Disease	Without Disease					
SI							
Disease nonspecific (Beccati et al,[28] 2011)	64	94	Completely distended SI loops, 58	83	85	85	83
Obstruction (Busoni et al,[5] 2011)	10	26	Dilated, turgid SI loops, 8	80	96	89	93
Strangulating obstruction (Klohnen et al,[1] 1996)	46	180	Amotile SI, 46	100	100	100	100
Strangulating obstruction (Klohnen et al,[1] 1996)	ND	ND	Abnormal SI wall thickness & distension, ND	98	84	62	99
Colic (Scharner et al,[27] 2015)	69	171	Decreased motility, wall thickening, 62	97 90–100[a]	93 88–96[a]	85 75–92[a]	99 96–100[a]
Inflammatory bowel disease (Ceriotti et al,[22] 1996)	19	16	Thickened SI ≥5.7 mm, ND	37	88	—	—
Ascarid infection (Nielsen et al,[26] 2016)	5	4	Scoring system, 5	100 48–100[a]	50 8–92[a]	71.4 29–96[a]	100 19–100[a]
Surgical need (Busoni et al,[5] 2011)	13	23	Dilated, turgid SI loops, 8	62	96	89	81
LC							
LCV							
Pease et al,[10] 2004	12	28	Thickened LC >9 mm, 8	67 36–98[a]	100 98–100[a]	100 94–100[a]	88 74–100[a]

(continued on next page)

Table 2
(continued)

Condition	Number of Cases With Disease	Number of Cases Without Disease	Measured Variable (n)	SN (%)	SP (%)	PPV (%)	NPV %
Beccati et al,[28] 2011	9	149	Thickened LC >5 mm, 22	67	86	87	97
			Absent motility, ND	63	77	77	96
Scharner et al,[27] 2015	19	231	Wall thickening, 12	63 38–84[a]	99 98–100[a]	92 36–100[a]	97 90–97[a]
RDDLC & 180° LCV Ness etal,[8] 2012	34	48	Visualized colonic mesenteric vessels, 24	68 52–83[a]	98 94–100[a]	96 88–100[a]	81 71–92[a]
RDDLC Scharner et al,[27] 2015	52	188	Horizontally running colonic vessels, 5	8.8 3–19[a]	100.0 98–100[a]	100.0 48–100[a]	77.9 72–83[a]
LDDLC Beccati et al,[28] 2011	16	142	No visualization of L kidney, 32	87	83	42	98
LDDLC Scharner et al,[27] 2015	11	229	No recognition of L kidney, 10	91 59–100[a]	98 95–99[a]	67 38–88[a]	99,6 98–100[a]
Sand impaction Korolainen & Ruohoniemi,[20] 2002	24	8	Grading system, 21	88 ±12%[a]	88 ±7%[a]	—	—
LC impaction (ingesta) Scharner et al,[27] 2015	47	193	Loss of normal position, poor motility, 14	29.8 17–45[a]	97 93–99[a]	70 46–88[a]	85 80–90[a]

Abbreviations: L, left; LC, large colon; LCV, large colon volvulus; LDDLC, left dorsal displacement of the large colon; ND, not discernible from report; NPP, negative predictive value; PPV, positive predictive value; RDDLC, right dorsal displacement of the large colon; SN, sensitivity; SP, specificity.
[a] 95% CI.

shadow and ventral displacement of the dorsal image of the splenic parenchyma. A diagnosis of lateral displacement was made if the entire image of the spleen was obliterated by gas or if the colon was fluid filled and transmitted US waves so that the colon, spleen, and kidney could be visualized. The inability to image the left kidney was considered supportive but not diagnostic. The investigators described this finding as being inconsistent and being reported in horses without clinical signs of colic.[30] Additionally, they described that an image of the left kidney can be obtained in some horses with NSE if the entrapped colon is free of gas and the colon caudal to the kidney contains ingesta.[29]

Forty-seven horses included in the study were determined to have LDDLC, but no reference standard was described. Fifteen horses had ultrasonographic results confirmed on celiotomy.[29] No false-positive findings were described, but false-negative results occurred in 5 horses.[29] The investigators discussed that this occurred in the first 10 months of a 28-month study and was likely a result of operator inexperience (observer bias).[29]

Despite the inability to image the left kidney not being considered diagnostic by the aforementioned study, it forms the standardized measurement in 2 subsequent studies.[27,28] These subsequent studies report a high number of false positives (n = 18)[28] and 5 false positives and 1 false negative.[27] These values account for the lower PPVs from these studies.

One study also reports rectal examination as less sensitive than ultrasonography in accuracy for LDDLC (72% vs 90%).[27]

Large Colon Volvulus

Venous occlusion that occurs during strangulating obstruction leads to the large colon wall becoming edematous and thickened.

Two studies state that a sensitivity of 67% is high for a thickened large colon as a test for large colon volvulus (LCV).[10,28] One study found a significant correlation between wall thickness with strangulating LCV but not nonstrangulating LCV.[28] However, this study identified a thickened large colon in 22 horses, with only 9 having a definitive diagnosis of strangulating LVC; it is not clear in the study how the false positives were accounted for. Another study obtained similar results.[27] The same study states that absent motility of the LCV had good sensitivity, specificity, and high NPV for both strangulating and nonstrangulating LCV.[28]

The rectal examination was also less sensitive in accuracy for large colon torsion (26% vs 63%).[27]

Right Dorsal Displacement of the Large Colon

The presence of normally medially situated mesenteric colonic vessels of the large colon, in the lateral cranial region of the right abdomen, has been assessed as an indicator that the bowel is in an abnormal position, as in an right dorsal displacement of the large colon (RDDLC) or 180 LCVs.[8] The investigators of this study regard this test as highly specific and moderately sensitive.[8] Another report describes this finding in 13 of 23 horses with a diagnosis of RDDLC at the exploratory laparotomy.[31] Statistics describing the accuracy of ultrasonography as a diagnostic test were not performed in this study. The investigators discuss that correct diagnosis by US of this condition depends in part on the type of RDDLC and the exact location in which the bowel is situated. A very low sensitivity (9% [95% CI = 3%–19%]) for the detection of large colon displacements in 57 horses with this disease, but a high specificity (100% [95% CI = 98%–100%]) based on not having any false-positive findings with this method, was reported from a different study. In this study, rectal examination had a far greater sensitivity for this disease 96% (95% CI = 88%–100%), with an also high specificity 89% (95% CI = 85%–93%).[27]

Impaction

The diagnosis of sand impaction with ultrasonography was compared with the results of radiographs.[20] Ultrasonography was reported to be a good method for detecting sand accumulations but was not as good as radiology.[20] For detecting impactions of ingesta in the large colon using ultrasonography, a low sensitivity (30% [17%–45%]) was obtained.[27] The specificity (97%; 93%–99%) was high, however, indicating that a positive test result would be useful at ruling in the disease.[27] The PPV and NPV were 70% (46%–88%) and 85% (80%–89%), respectively. The investigators of the aforementioned study conclude that although ultrasonography helps better identify severe diseases of the GI tract and should be included in the routine examination of horses with colic, the technique does not replace the rectal examination, which is superior in the diagnosis of large colon displacements and impactions.

Other Gastrointestinal Accuracy Studies

To study the effect of test results on clinical decisions, an attempt to look at whether the FLASH ultrasonographic technique was accurate for predicting surgical need was made.[5] Low numbers were included in the study, and several false-positive test results lowered the specificity and predictive values.[5] The low sensitivity for surgical need is explained as being from 5 horses out of 13 undergoing surgery that had false-negative results on the US.

Additional studies of clinical decision-making could provide information on whether the sonographic information would change a treatment plan in patients.

SUMMARY

This article reviews ultrasonographic techniques for the diagnosis of diseases of the equine GI tract. Many diseases of the GI tract have used US examination as part of the diagnostic process. Accuracy studies are reviewed, and clear reporting of results are necessary to assess the usefulness of ultrasonography as a diagnostic test in clinical practice. Ultrasonography seems to be most accurate in diagnosing severe SI lesions. Additional studies, as outlined, would be necessary to provide more information on the usefulness of ultrasonography in managing clinical cases.

REFERENCES

1. Klohnen A, Vachon AM, Fischer AT. Use of diagnostic ultrasonography in horses with signs of acute abdominal pain. J Am Vet Med Assoc 1996;209(9):1597–601.
2. Reef VB, Whittier M, Allam L. Sonographic evaluation of the adult abdomen. Clin Tech Equine Pract 2004;3(3):294–307.
3. McAuliffe SB. Abdominal ultrasonography of the foal. Clin Tech Equine Pract 2004;3(3):308–16.
4. Porter M, Ramirez S. Equine neonatal thoracic and abdominal ultrasonography. Vet Clin North Am Equine Pract 2005;21(2):407–29.
5. Busoni V, De Busscher V, Lopez D, et al. Evaluation of a protocol for fast localised abdominal sonography of horses (FLASH) admitted for colic. Vet J 2011;188(1): 77–82.
6. Williams S, Cooper J, Freeman S. Evaluation of normal findings using a detailed and focused technique for transcutaneous abdominal ultrasonography in the horse. BMC Vet Res 2014;10(Suppl 1):S5.

7. Abutarbush SM. Use of ultrasonography to diagnose large colon volvulus in horses. J Am Vet Med Assoc 2006;228(3):409–13.

8. Ness SL, Bain FT, Zantingh AJ, et al. Ultrasonographic visualization of colonic mesenteric vasculature as an indicator of large colon right dorsal displacement or 180° volvulus (or both) in horses. Can Vet J 2012;53(4):378–82.

9. Le Jeune S, Whitcomb MB. Ultrasound of the equine acute abdomen. Vet Clin North Am Equine Pract 2014;30(2):353–81.

10. Pease A, Scrivani P, Erb H, et al. Accuracy of increased large-intestine wall thickness during ultrasonography for diagnosing large-colon torsion in 42 horses. Vet Radiol Ultrasound 2004;45(3):220–4.

11. Silva CT, Daneman A, Navarro OM, et al. A prospective comparison of intestinal sonography and abdominal radiographs in a neonatal intensive care unit. Pediatr Radiol 2013;43(11):1453–63.

12. Aleman M, Gillis CL, Nieto JE. Ultrasonographic anatomy and biometric analysis of the thoracic and abdominal organs in healthy foals from birth to age 6 months. Equine Vet J 2002;34(7):649–55.

13. Kirberger R, van den Berg J, Gottschalk R, et al. Duodenal ultrasonography in the normal adult horse. Vet Radiol Ultrasound 1995;36(1):50–6.

14. Epstein K, Short D, Parente E, et al. Gastrointestinal ultrasonography in normal adult ponies. Vet Radiol Ultrasound 2008;49(3):282–6.

15. Freeman S. Ultrasonography of the equine abdomen: findings in the colic patient. In Pract 2002;24(5):262–73.

16. Magee AA, Ragle CA, Hines MT, et al. Anorectal lymphadenopathy causing colic, perirectal abscesses, or both in five young horses. J Am Vet Med Assoc 1997; 210(6):804–7.

17. Torkelson J. Perirectal abscess, colic, and dyschezia in a horse. Can Vet J 2002; 43(2):127.

18. Bossuyt PM, Reitsma JB, Bruns DE, et al. Towards complete and accurate reporting of studies of diagnostic accuracy: the STARD initiative. 2003. Clin Chem Lab Med 2003;41(1):68–73.

19. Hulley SB, Cummings SR, Browner WS, et al. Designing clinical research. 2nd edition. Philadelphia: Lippincott Williams & Wilkins; 2013. p. 37–49.

20. Korolainen R, Ruohoniemi M. Reliability of ultrasonography compared to radiography in revealing intestinal sand accumulations in horses. Equine Vet J 2002; 34(5):499–504.

21. Ruohoniemi M, Kaikkonen R, Raekallio M, et al. Abdominal radiography in monitoring the resolution of sand accumulations from the large colon of horses treated medically. Equine Vet J 2001;33(1):59–64.

22. Ceriotti S, Zucca E, Stancari G, et al. Sensitivity and specificity of ultrasonographic evaluation of small intestine wall thickness in the diagnosis of inflammatory bowel disease in horses: a retrospective study. J Equine Vet Sci 2016;37:6–10.

23. Lindberg R, Nygren A, Persson S. Rectal biopsy diagnosis in horses with clinical signs of intestinal disorders: a retrospective study of 116 cases. Equine Vet J 1996;28(4):275–84.

24. Altman DG, Bland JM. Diagnostic tests. 1: sensitivity and specificity. BMJ 1994; 308(6943):1552.

25. Altman DG, Bland JM. Diagnostic tests 2: predictive values. BMJ 1994; 309(6947):102.

26. Nielsen MK, Donoghue EM, Stephens ML, et al. An ultrasonographic scoring method for transabdominal monitoring of ascarid burdens in foals. Equine Vet J 2016;48(3):380–6.

27. Scharner D, Bankert J, Brehm W. Comparison of the findings of rectal examination and ultrasonographic findings in horses with colic. Tierarztl Prax Ausg G Grosstiere Nutztiere 2015;43(5):278–86 [in German].

28. Beccati F, Pepe M, Gialletti R, et al. Is there a statistical correlation between ultrasonographic findings and definitive diagnosis in horses with acute abdominal pain? Equine Vet J Suppl 2011;39:98–105.

29. Santschi EM, Slone DE, Frank WM. Use of ultrasound in horses for diagnosis of left dorsal displacement of the large colon and monitoring its nonsurgical correction. Vet Surg 1993;22(4):281–4.

30. Rantanan NW. Diseases of the abdomen. Vet Clin North Am Equine Pract 1986;2:67–88.

31. Grenager NS, Durham MG. Ultrasonographic evidence of colonic mesenteric vessels as an indicator of right dorsal displacement of the large colon in 13 horses. Equine Vet J Suppl 2011;(39):153–5.

Diagnosis and Treatment of Undifferentiated and Infectious Acute Diarrhea in the Adult Horse

Sarah D. Shaw, DVM[a,b,1], Henry Stämpfli, DVM, Dr Med Vet[b,*]

KEYWORDS

- Equine • Colitis • Typhlocolitis • Infectious diarrhea • Intravenous fluid therapy

KEY POINTS

- Strict biosecurity measures should be enforced for all cases of acute diarrhea in adult horses.
- Diagnostic tests for salmonellosis, clostridiosis, coronavirus, and Potomac horse fever are evolving.
- Aims of treatment of acute diarrhea include fluid resuscitation, correction of electrolyte abnormalities, and limiting the systemic inflammatory response.
- Limited evidence exists to support many of the medications used to treat acute diarrhea and the judicious use of therapeutics is warranted.

INTRODUCTION

Acute diarrhea associated with colitis or typhlocolitis is a major cause of morbidity in horses and is life-threatening. Clinical signs of colic, hypovolemia, and endotoxemia result from altered motility, hypersecretion of fluid, and disruption of the mucosal barrier secondary to intestinal inflammation.

Undifferentiated and infectious acute diarrhea is a diagnostic and therapeutic challenge. Differential diagnoses for the acutely diarrheic horse share similar clinical and clinicopathologic features. Determination of causation is rarely possible. The fundamental diagnostic approach includes assessment of hydration, electrolyte and

[a] Rotenberg Veterinary P.C., Palgrave, Ontario LOG 1WO, Canada; [b] Large Animal Medicine, Department of Clinical Studies, Ontario Veterinary College, University of Guelph, Guelph, Ontario N1G 2W1, Canada
[1] Present address: PO Box 1015, Tottenham, Ontario L0G 1W0, Canada.
* Corresponding author. Department of Clinical Studies, Ontario Veterinary College, University of Guelph, 50 Stoneroad, Guelph, Ontario N1G 2W1, Canada.
E-mail address: hstaempf@uoguelph.ca

Vet Clin Equine 34 (2018) 39–53
https://doi.org/10.1016/j.cveq.2017.11.002
0749-0739/18/© 2017 Elsevier Inc. All rights reserved.
vetequine.theclinics.com

acid-base abnormalities, mucosal integrity, organ function, and the inflammatory response. Immediate therapeutic intervention, often in the absence of a definitive diagnosis, reduces comorbidities and mortality.

INITIAL DIAGNOSTICS
Bloodwork

Hematologic abnormalities seen early in the course of gastrointestinal disease reflect stress and endotoxemia. Leukopenia may be characterized by lymphopenia, neutropenia with or without a left shift, and toxic changes in neutrophils. A neutrophilic leukocytosis may be seen later. Degenerative left shifts and the presence of metamyelocytes and myelocytes are poor prognostic indicators.[1] Hemoconcentration and thrombocytopenia are common. Horses with a packed cell volume greater than 45% were 3.5 times less likely to survive.[2] Hyperfibrinogenemia and elevated serum amyloid A may be seen in acute, severe, colitis[3]

Diarrhea in horses is associated with hemodynamic and electrolyte changes caused by intraluminal sequestration of fluid. Serum biochemistry often reveals renal or prerenal azotemia and electrolyte abnormalities including hyponatremia, hypochloremia, hypokalemia, and hypocalcemia. In one retrospective, negative base excess was the best prognostic indicator.[4] In a study of 101 horses, plasma lactate at admission was not associated with survival status. However, reduction in serial lactate concentration by greater than or equal to 30% 4 to 8 hours and by greater than or equal to 50% 24 hours after admission was significantly associated with survival.[5] A creatinine concentration greater than 2.0 mg/dL (176.8 μmol/L) was also associated with a lower likelihood of survival.[2] Hyperproteinemia may be present with severe dehydration, although mild to severe hypoproteinemia is also seen as a result of gastrointestinal protein loss.

Ultrasonography

Abdominal ultrasonography is an important diagnostic aid in cases of acute diarrhea and should be performed to assess large and small intestinal wall thickness and peritoneal fluid volume and character. See Nicola C. Cribb, Luis G. Arroyo's article, "Techniques and Accuracy of Abdominal Ultrasound in Gastro-Intestinal Diseases of Horses and Foals," in this issue for more details.

Pathogen-Specific Serologic and Fecal Diagnostics

Commercial laboratories frequently offer diarrhea panels, which are helpful for screening for numerous pathogens. However, like any screening test, specificity may be compromised and results should be interpreted with caution. Furthermore, some diagnostic laboratories include tests that are unnecessary or not clinically relevant in the adult horse. **Table 1** provides a summary of commercially available fecal and serologic diagnostics and their limitations.

DIFFERENTIAL DIAGNOSES
Salmonellosis

Salmonellosis is a well-recognized cause of acute diarrhea in the horse. It is reported as a result of infection with Salmonella enterica subsp. enterica, a G⁻, facultative anaerobic bacterium. Numerous serovars are associated with clinical disease but Salmonella typhimurium is commonly isolated from diarrheic horses and associated with high pathogenicity.[6] Salmonella infection in adult horses ranges from the inapparent carrier state, to pyrexia, anorexia, leukopenia, and depression without diarrhea, to acute, severe, enterocolitis with diarrhea.

Table 1
Diagnostic tests for acute diarrhea in the adult horse

Pathogen	Diagnostic Tests	Comments
Salmonella *spp*	Fecal PCR	Potentially highly sensitive and specific. Fast turnaround time. Serial samples needed.
	Fecal culture	Slower but provides isolates for susceptibility testing and typing. Serial samples needed. Sensitivity is impacted greatly by laboratory methods, such as enrichment culture, and laboratory experience.
Clostridium difficile	Culture (isolation with selective media)	Extra testing required to determine if isolates are toxigenic.
	Antigen ELISA	Quick and inexpensive. Very sensitive but lower specificity. Will detect toxigenic and nontoxigenic strains. Most often used as in initial screening test because of high negative predictive value, with positives tested by ELISA or PCR.
	Toxin A/B II ELISA, (or cytopathic effect cell culture)	Performance of different commercial assays on horse feces is likely highly variable. Has been clinical standard for diagnosis.
	PCR for TcdA and TcdB	Can be quick and highly sensitive. False-positives can occur because of detection of carriers, which is common in some populations.
Clostridium perfringens	Culture	Low diagnostic yield because of common shedding by healthy horses.
	Culture + PCR	PCR to detect selected toxin genes can increase diagnostic relevance, particularly with genes more commonly associated with disease (eg, NetF, beta2).
	Toxin-ELISA	Currently restricted to enterotoxin. Positive results are suggestive but enterotoxin is detected in some healthy horses.
	PCR	Genotyping is available in specialized laboratories.
Coronavirus	Fecal PCR	Epidemiology of ECoV is not well established but positive results in horses with disease consistent with ECoV infection provides a presumptive diagnosis.
Neorickettsia risticii	Fecal and blood PCR	Detection in blood may be more sensitive early in the course of disease; horses become PCR positive on feces later.
	Serology (IFA)	Single serum samples are not diagnostic.

Abbreviations: ECoV, equine coronavirus; ELISA, enzyme-linked immunosorbent assay; IFA, indirect fluorescent antibody; PCR, polymerase chain reaction; TcdA, *C difficile* toxin A; TcdB, *C difficile* are toxin B.

Clinically apparent salmonellosis in adult horses most commonly manifests as enterocolitis with large-volume, watery diarrhea with subsequent bacteremia.[7] Profound neutropenia is characteristic in *Salmonella* infections and results from neutrophil margination, invasion into the intestinal villi, and loss in the intestinal lumen.[8] Intestinal mucosal damage permits bacterial entry into the portal circulation, potentially damaging hepatocytes and increasing serum levels of sorbitol dehydrogenase and aspartate transaminase.[8] Dehydration is severe and is associated with prerenal azotemia and decreased blood pH. Clinical signs of pyrexia, inappetance, diarrhea, and colic are largely a result of the host inflammatory response.

Risk factors for infection include recent abdominal surgery, antimicrobial administration, transportation, gastrointestinal disease, immunosuppression, diet changes, respiratory disease, high ambient temperature, and general anesthesia.[9–11] Historically, a diagnosis of *Salmonella* colitis was made through identification of the organism on fecal culture, but it is only intermittently shed. Real-time quantitative polymerase chain reaction (qPCR) has largely replaced culture based on shorter time to results, increased relative sensitivity, and potentially fewer serial samples required to detect *Salmonella*.[7,12] Between three and five serial fecal samples (for PCR or culture), depending on laboratory methods, are recommended to determine negative *Salmonella* status.

Treatment in early disease is mainly supportive with intravenous, isotonic fluids directed at volume replacement and to buy time for tissue recovery. Acid-base and electrolyte abnormalities should be corrected and inflammation controlled. Severe leukopenia frequently occurs in cases of *Salmonella* infection and warrants consideration of antimicrobial therapy with aminoglycosides, fluoroquinolones, or cephalosporins. Given the propensity for this organism to cause microthrombosis and infarction, anticoagulant therapy may be considered. Nosocomial *Salmonella* infections and hospital biosecurity have been the focus of recent literature. Outbreaks in teaching hospitals have resulted in prolonged closures, significant economic losses, and decreased clinic time for veterinary students. Strict biosecurity measures should be enforced in cases of acute diarrhea to prevent the potential nosocomial spread of *Salmonella* spp and other highly infectious organisms.

Clostridiosis

Colitis as a result of *Clostridium difficile* infection (CDI) was first described in horses in 1987. *Clostridium perfringens* and *C difficile* are the clostridial species most commonly associated with diarrhea, with sporadic cases attributed to *Clostridium septicum*, *Clostridium sordelli*, and *Clostridium cadaveris*.

Clostridium difficile

C difficile is a common isolate in cases of colitis in adult horses. CDI has received recent attention in the human literature, although the most prevalent ribotypes responsible for disease differ between humans and animals. *C difficile* is isolated from the manure of healthy horses and prevalence rates range from 0% to 33%.[13,14] Thus, the carrier state in horses and livestock has been suggested as a reservoir for human CDI.

The most important risk factors for CDI in adult horses are antimicrobial administration and hospitalization. Isolation of toxigenic *C difficile* has been associated with the administration of all antimicrobials, most notably β-lactams, gentamicin, trimethoprim sulfonamides, clindamycin, erythromycin, and rifampicin.[14] Proton pump inhibitors and H_2 antagonists have been implicated in the development of CDI in horses, but strong evidence is lacking.

The most important virulence factors of *C difficile* are toxin A (TcdA, an enterotoxin) and toxin B (TcdB, a cytotoxin). Clinical disease, however, only occurs when the normal gastrointestinal flora is disrupted and toxigenic strains of *C difficile* proliferate. In humans CDI is acute or chronic, whereas chronic CDI in horses has not been described.

C difficile colitis varies from peracute colitis with a rapid decline to a milder, more prolonged course. Horses may be pyrexic, depressed, and anorexic before developing diarrhea and gastrointestinal signs. Neutropenia, hypoproteinemia, dehydration, hemoconcentration, and electrolyte and acid-base abnormalities may all be appreciated. *C difficile* is challenging to culture so false-negative test results are possible and CDI is therefore likely underdiagnosed. Enzyme immunoassays have been developed for the identification of TcdA and TcdB, although their performance is highly variable. More recently, molecular detection methods following bacterial culture have been used to identify genes for TcdA and TcdB in the feces of horses.[15,16]

Aside from supportive care, specific treatments for CDI remain controversial. Evidence exists that *Saccharomyces boulardii*, a nonpathogenic yeast, can destroy TcdA.[17] Di-tri-octahedral smectite binds TcdA and TcdB in a dose-dependent manner in vitro and may be useful to limit the toxemic effects of these toxins. Metronidazole is commonly used to treat *C difficile* colitis in horses to reduce the *C difficile* population, whereas the normal flora is restored. Although metronidazole resistance has been documented in cases of human infection, it is not a prevalent feature in equine CDI.[14] However, even targeted antimicrobial therapy can have deleterious effects on the microbiota and may disrupt or delay recolonization with beneficial bacteria. Recently, fecal transfaunation, also known as fecal microbial transplantation or fecal bacteriotherapy, has re-emerged as a treatment of CDI in humans and horses. Proximal duodenal infusion with donor feces was significantly more effective than standard vancomycin therapy in humans with recurrent CDI.[18] Anecdotal evidence supports the use of fecal microbial slurries via nasogastric intubation for treatment of acute cases of equine CDI.[19] Further investigation is needed to provide evidence-based support.

Clostridium perfringens

C perfringens is associated with occasional cases of acute diarrhea in adult horses. It has been isolated from the gastrointestinal flora of normal horses, although reported prevalence rates are low, ranging from 0% to 8% in healthy adult horses.[13] It is classified into five types (A to E) based on exotoxin production. *C perfringens* type A is the isolate most commonly cultured from healthy and diarrheic adult horses. β2 toxin, suspected to be produced by a subtype of *C perfringens* type A, has been associated with clinical *C perfringens* infections in horses with colitis.[20,21] β-toxin produced by types B and C has direct cytotoxic effects resulting in enterocyte necrosis, mucosal ulceration, and hemorrhagic diarrhea. Enterotoxin, produced by both type A and type C strains, creates pores and alters membrane permeability, leading to cell necrosis. The pore-forming toxin NetF has also been recently identified as a major virulence determinant and has been associated with necrotizing enteritis in foals and dogs.

Clinical signs of *C perfringens* vary from peracute fatal colitis to a milder presentation with anorexia, depression, and pyrexia. Gastrointestinal signs include profuse, watery diarrhea that may be hemorrhagic. Affected horses demonstrate nonspecific signs of colic, endotoxemia, and dehydration. Given its presence in the feces of normal horses, the diagnosis of *C perfringens* colitis is challenging. Quantitative fecal culture no longer supports a diagnosis of *C perfringens* colitis. Enzyme immunoassays for the *C perfringens* enterotoxin detect its presence in healthy and clinically affected horses. More recently, PCR has been used to detect toxin genes, although not proving a causal relation.[15] Therapy is mainly supportive. Specific therapy aimed at binding exotoxins includes treatment with di-tri-octahedral smectite.[22,23] There is limited evidence of the benefits of metronidazole therapy in cases of *C perfringens* colitis.

Coronavirus

Equine coronavirus (ECoV) has recently emerged as a significant enteric pathogen in adult horses.[24,25] Although coronaviruses have been long identified in the feces of adult horses and foals, their role in the pathogenesis of enteric fever and diarrhea was only recently elucidated after outbreaks of clinical disease. ECoV is an enveloped, positive-stranded RNA virus belonging to the Betacoronavirus-1 genus. Transmission is believed to be via the fecal-oral route. Infection begins in the small intestine. Lesions include necrosis and sloughing of enterocytes in the intestinal villi, dilated crypts filled with necrotic debris, and mucosal inflammation.[25,26]

Hematologic abnormalities include leukopenia, characterized by neutropenia and/or lymphopenia.[25] The most common clinical manifestations of ECoV infection include anorexia, lethargy, and fever.[22,25] In a report of 59 clinical cases, diarrhea and colic were only seen 20% and 7% of affected horses, respectively.[25] Neurologic signs associated with ECoV infection have been described and seem to be associated with hyperammonemic encephalopathy with Alzheimer type II astrocytosis in the cerebral cortex.[26]

Diagnosis of ECoV colitis is currently based on PCR of feces, gastrointestinal contents, or tissue samples. In one study there was no significant statistical difference in absolute ECoV quantification between positive sick and positive healthy horses. However, the overall agreement between clinical status (horses demonstrating clinical signs of ECoV infection) and ECoV-positive status on PCR was 91%.[25] Therapy is directed at supportive care and prevention of hyperammonemic encephalopathy.

Potomac Horse Fever

Potomac horse fever (PHF), or equine neorickettsiosis, was first recognized as a cause of acute typhlocolitis in horses in the United States in 1984 along the Potomac River area and has since been described in Canada, Uruguay, Brazil, and Europe. This acute, potentially fatal disease is an infection with the gram-negative, obligate, intracellular, bacterial endosymbiont *Neorickettsia risticii*.[27] The bacterium survives in digenic trematodes, such as *Acanthatrium* and *Lecithodendrium* spp.[28] Trematodes use freshwater and lymnaeid snails as first intermediate hosts and aquatic insects (mayflies, caddisflies, damselflies, dragonflies, and stoneflies) as second intermediate hosts.[29,30] The definitive hosts of these trematodes are brown bats (*Eptesicus fuscus* and *Myotis lucifugus*). Horses become accidental hosts of digenic trematodes when they inadvertently ingest infected intermediate hosts. *N risticii* is released from the trematode and once inside the equine gastrointestinal tract it invades and replicates within the colonic epithelial cells. It also translocates into blood monocytes (equine monocytic ehrlichiosis), mast cells, and tissue macrophages. A seasonal rise in disease incidence is seen during warmer months.

The most common clinical signs of PHF are diarrhea, fever, anorexia, depression, and colic.[30] Abortions may also occur as a result of *N risticii* infection. In one retrospective of 44 horses with PHF, laminitis was identified in 36%, of which 88% were affected in all four feet.[30] Horses present with clinicopathologic abnormalities typically seen in equine colitis. The same study identified that serum creatinine and urea nitrogen concentrations, hematocrit, red blood count, blood hemoglobin concentration, band neutrophils, serum aspartate transaminase, serum CK, and anion gap were significantly higher in nonsurvivors. Further, serum chloride, serum sodium, and duration of hospitalization were significantly lower in nonsurvivors.[30]

Diagnostics for PHF include serum indirect fluorescent antibody testing, enzyme-linked immunosorbent assay, culture of *N risticii* from buffy coat or feces, and PCR on whole blood or feces. Both exposure and vaccination lead to many false positives with antibody testing and in one study 16% of healthy horses had a rise in paired indirect fluorescent antibody titers,[31] so antigen testing is recommended. Culture of *N risticii* remains the gold standard of diagnosis, although PCR was reported to identify 81% of culture-positive, naturally infected horses.[32]

Tetracycline antibiotics effectively kill *N risticii* and oxytetracycline administration to horses with clinical signs of disease has been positively associated with survival.[30] Additional therapy is supportive and includes fluid replacement and laminitis prevention. Particular attention should be paid to fluid resuscitation in hypovolemic horses either before, or in conjunction with, administration of nephrotoxic drugs (oxytetracycline and nonsteroidal anti-inflammatory drugs [NSAIDs]). Several killed and adjuvants vaccines have been marketed. However, vaccine failure rates are high,[33,34] likely caused by the antigenic differences present among greater than 14 *N rickettsia* strains isolated from clinical cases.[27]

TREATMENT AND SUPPORTIVE CARE
Fluid Therapy

Fluid therapy in gastrointestinal disease has been covered in depth.[35] Fluid plans should be based on clinical and clinicopathologic assessment. Fluid deficits are based on the formula:

Volume deficit (L) = Bwt (kg) $*$ % dehydration

A generally accepted approach is replacement of the volume deficit at a rate of 10 to 20 mL/kg/h.[35] The patient should be reassessed every 4 to 6 hours and changes to the fluid plan made according to changes in hydration status. Maintenance requirements and ongoing fluid losses should also be calculated to administer fluids at an appropriate rate:

Maintenance fluid volume = 50 to 100 mL/kg per 24 hours

The goal of fluid therapy is volume resuscitation and correction of lactic acidosis; commercially available, balanced, isotonic fluids should be administered. Fluid supplementation decisions should be made based on serum electrolytes and acid-base status. Lactic acidosis caused by dehydration is common. Hypokalemia is common in anorectic horses with gastrointestinal disease and should be addressed when serum potassium is less than 3 mEq/L. Sodium bicarbonate supplementation is considered if the base deficit is greater than -10 mEq/L or the pH is less than 7.2. The required amount of sodium bicarbonate should be administered as an isotonic solution over a period of 24 hours.[35] It is important to remember that the administration of sodium bicarbonate does not correct a metabolic acidosis (lactic acidosis) secondary to dehydration. Therefore, sodium bicarbonate should be used as adjunct therapy to balanced isotonic fluids, and only if metabolic acidosis is severe. The amount of sodium bicarbonate required is estimated using the following formula:

$Na-HCO_3$ (mmoL/L) = BE x BW x 0.3

An ionized calcium level of less than 1.4 mg/dL (0.3493 mmol/L)[35] and decreased intestinal motility are indications for calcium supplementation.

Colloid Oncotic Support

The general indications for the use of colloids include hypovolemia, hypoproteinemia, and decreased osmotic pressure. Because hypoproteinemia is common in horses with diarrhea, synthetic colloids and commercial equine plasma are often administered.

The literature evaluating the use of synthetic colloids in horses is limited to experimental studies and small population clinical evaluations. Hydroxyethyl starch (HES) increased colloid osmotic pressure (COP) in normal ponies but had dose-dependent effects on hemostatic variables, leading a trend in prolongation of bleeding times.[36] In hypoproteinemic horses, HES had a modest effect on COP but administering typical doses did not restore COP to normal.[37,38] In an experimental endotoxemia, the use of HES with hypertonic saline solution exerted no benefit on cardiac output or systemic vascular resistance compared with isotonic fluid resuscitation.[39] Furthermore, no significant differences in coagulation measures were noted between horses treated with HES versus isotonic fluids.[40] However, HES has been shown to adversely affect platelet function in vitro and in healthy horses.[41,42]

The use of synthetic colloids over crystalloids in human patients with sepsis has been questioned. Colloid administration has been associated with acute kidney injury, osmotic nephrosis, hemorrhage, anaphylactoid reactions, tissue accumulation, hepatic organ failure, and pruritus. Despite numerous randomized clinical trials and meta-analyses, there is conflicting evidence correlating colloid administration with increased mortality rates and increased need for renal-replacement therapy. However, the 2012 Surviving Sepsis Campaign recommended against the use of HES in sepsis.[43] As a result, the European Medicine Agency concluded that HES solutions should not be used in patients with sepsis or critically ill patients and the Food and Drug Administration placed a boxed warning on HES for increased mortality and renal-replacement therapy in 2013.

A recent study comparing the effects of HES versus commercial equine plasma on clinicopathologic values and COP in healthy horses revealed both products produced equivalent, although modest, increases in plasma COP. Meanwhile, plasma had a less profound and less prolonged dilutional effect on hematocrit, blood hemoglobin, serum total protein, and albumin concentration compared with HES.[44]

The benefits of HES over plasma include lower cost, easier storage, higher oncotic pressure, and no risk of infectious disease transmission.[44] However, equine plasma provides immunoglobulins, coagulation factors, and antithrombin. Plasma may also be less likely to result in acute kidney injury or coagulation abnormalities in critically ill patients. Although evidence from the human literature cannot be applied to equine medicine, there is a need for further evaluation of HES use in critically ill and septic horses. In the meantime, judicious use of colloids in these patients is recommended.

Antimicrobial Therapy

The advantages and disadvantages of antimicrobial administration should be considered before use in cases of acute diarrhea. In one retrospective, horses presenting with colitis that were previously treated with antimicrobials were 4.5 times less likely to survive than those not treated.[2] Antimicrobial use affects the fecal microbiota,[45,46] which is likely already disturbed.[47] Procaine penicillin, ceftiofur sodium, and trimethoprim sulfadiazine administration all impacted the fecal microbiota in healthy horses, and changes often persisted for 25 days.[46]

The identification or clinical suspicion of the presence of certain pathogens warrants targeted antimicrobial use. Oxytetracycline is considered the treatment of choice for horses with PHF.[30] Metronidazole is recommended for the treatment of C difficile–associated diarrhea (CDAD) in humans and is often used to treat horses with confirmed or presumed CDAD. However, Magdesian and colleagues[15] demonstrated an association between metronidazole administration and identification of metronidazole-resistant C difficile strains. Although metronidazole resistance in horses with CDIs is not considered clinically important at this time, these strains are suspected to be more virulent.[14] To this effect, horses with metronidazole-resistant strains of *C difficile* had an increased risk of mortality compared with horses infected with metronidazole-susceptible strains.[15]

Antimicrobial therapy may be warranted in acute diarrhea cases demonstrating severe neutropenia and/or evidence of septic foci, such as in the lungs, liver, or jugular veins. Antimicrobial drug selection should be based on culture and susceptibility patterns of the causative agents whenever possible. However, in cases of acute undifferentiated diarrhea in horses, antibiotics may be contraindicated because of further disruption of the microbiota. Furthermore, increased shedding of *Salmonella* was associated with the administration of antimicrobials[48] and multidrug resistance in *Salmonella* spp is an emerging threat. Therefore, judicious use of systemic antimicrobials is strongly recommended.

Limiting the Effects of Endotoxemia

Efforts should be made to limit endotoxin entry into circulation, reduce the release of inflammatory mediators, neutralize circulating endotoxin, and provide supportive care.[49] NSAIDs inhibit cyclooxygenase enzymes associated with early hemodynamic responses to endotoxin. Both flunixin meglumine and ketoprofen significantly decreased the production of thromboxane B_2 production by blood monocytes in vitro.[50] Low doses of flunixin meglumine (0.25 mg/kg) suppressed thromboxane and prostaglandin production in horses challenged with endotoxin.[51] Although a dose of 1.1 mg/kg is also antiendotoxic, the lower dose may be associated with fewer side effects, especially in cases with renal insufficiency. Administration of NSAIDs to horses with endotoxemia is a mainstay of treatment. Albeit in practice, treatment is initiated following challenge with endogenous endotoxins, whereas experimentally, benefits were noted when NSAIDs were administered before endotoxin exposure. Clinicians often administer flunixin meglumine every 8 hours to control the clinical signs of endotoxemia while limiting adverse side effects, such as renal papillary necrosis and gastrointestinal ulceration.[49]

Polymyxin B is a cationic polypeptide antibiotic that forms a stable complex with the lipid A component of lipopolysaccharide. Once bound, lipopolysaccharide does not interact with equine inflammatory cells, thus preventing initiation of the proinflammatory cascade.[49,52] Initial high doses reportedly produced signs of neurotoxicity and nephrotoxicity. When administered to healthy horses at doses between 1000 and 5000 IU/kg, polymyxin B inhibited 75% of endotoxin-induced tumor necrosis factor activity[53] and no alterations in either creatinine[53] nor urine γ-glutamyltransferase-to-creatinine ratios[52] were noted. However, polymyxin B should be used with caution in hypovolemic and azotemic animals and should always be administered diluted in isotonic fluids. If side effects of neuromuscular blockage or other neurologic side effects occur, administration should be discontinued.

Hyperimmune plasma or serum, derived from horses immunized against G-bacteria and endotoxin, has the proposed benefits of neutralizing endotoxin and modulating leukocyte activation. However, there is conflicting evidence of the benefits of administration of hyperimmune plasma in experimental models of endotoxemia in horses.[49] A recent study[54] revealed that pretreatment with hyperimmune equine plasma failed to modify clinical signs of experimentally induced endotoxemia and had no impact on leukocyte activation, but reduced the bioactivity of tumor necrosis factor-α. Further studies are needed to evaluate the clinical benefits of hyperimmune plasma or serum in endotoxemic horses.

Pentoxifylline is a methyxanthine derivative that increases the deformability of red blood cells, suppresses production of proinflammatory cytokines, and can inhibit the activation of B and T cells.[55] Experimentally, pentoxifylline administration had limited beneficial effects in endotoxemic horses[56] and slight benefits in combination therapy with flunixin meglumine.[57] Pentoxifylline is most commonly used in horses with laminitis and placentitis to increase microvascular blood flow, but there are currently no published controlled clinical trials supporting its use.

Intraluminal Intestinal Binding Agents

In theory, binding exotoxins and endotoxin within the gut lumen may decrease systemic absorption in horses with colitis. Di-tri-octaheadral smectite is a negatively charged, hydrated, aluminomagnesium that binds positively charged organic cations. Dose-dependent binding of Di-tri-octaheadral smectite with C difficile toxins A and B, C perfringens enterotoxin, and endotoxin has been demonstrated in vitro.[23,24] The recommended dose is a 1.4-kg loading dose followed by 454 g every 6 to 12 hours, necessitating frequent nasogastric intubation. Activated charcoal is a nonspecific binding agent used in many monogastric species. A recent in vitro study demonstrated no significant effects of activated charcoal on the microbial population, major metabolites produced, rate of gas production, or pH values.[58] These findings suggest that the impact of activated charcoal on the equine hindgut, and binding of toxic substances, may be minimal. Further in vivo studies are needed to elucidate the benefits of these binding agents.

Probiotics

Probiotics are discussed elsewhere in this issue. In one study of 14 horses with diarrhea, administration of S boulardii decreased the duration of diarrhea from 7 to 5 days, compared with control horses.[59] In contrast, there was no significant difference in return to normal manure, return to normal heart rate, appetite improvement, or any other clinical variables measured between Saccharomyces-treated and control horses in a randomized prospective study.[60]

The administration of Lactobacillillus spp and Bifidobacterium animalis lactis had no impact on clostridial shedding and minimal impact on the composition of the fecal microbiota in foals when administered for 3 weeks.[61] Recent literature suggests that orally administered probiotics (Pediococcus acidilactici and S boulardii) may have immunomodulatory effects in horses.[62] At this time, there is conflicting evidence regarding the clinical benefit of probiotic administration. Furthermore, label claims on veterinary probiotic preparations often contain gross inaccuracies and quality control of products is lacking.[63,64]

Additional Supportive Care Measures

Gastroprotectants such as omeprazole and H_2 antagonists, are often used prophylactically to prevent gastric ulceration in anorectic horses with acute diarrhea. Proton pump inhibitor administration has long been suspected to be a risk factor for CDAD in humans, although high-quality evidence of a cause-effect relationship is lacking.[65] Foals treated with antiulcer medication were two times more likely to develop diarrhea than those left untreated, but this was not associated with CDI.[66] The relationship between antiulcer medications, diarrhea, and CDAD in adult horses is unknown, but increasing gastric pH may eliminate a defense against C difficile and other pathogens.

Laminitis is commonly encountered in cases of sepsis. Currently, distal limb cryotherapy (applied from hoof to carpus for 72 hours continuously) is the only method of prevention of laminitis in horses with systemic inflammation that has been validated.[67] Other feasible laminitis prevention techniques include treating the primary disease process, anti-inflammatory therapy (NSAIDs, pentoxifylline), inhibition of neutrophil and platelet margination (low-molecular-weight heparin, pentoxifylline, aspirin, and possibly corticosteroids), antioxidant therapy (dimethyl sulfoxide), and physical support of the sole with easing of breakover.[68]

Bacterial sepsis has the potential to lead to disseminated intravascular coagulation secondary to widespread inflammation. Salmonellosis has been associated with thrombotic events in ewes and disseminated intravascular coagulation in horses.[8] In a controlled clinical trial in humans with sepsis, heparin improved hypercoagulable states, reduced time in the intensive care unit, and decreased days on mechanical ventilation.[69] In a retrospective study of 360 horses that underwent colic surgery, the prevalence and grade of laminitis was lower in horses treated with low-molecular-weight heparin.[70] Although unfractioned heparin is often used for prophylaxis of coagulation disorders, low-molecular-weight heparin was associated with fewer side effects, such as decreased packed cell volume (PCV), catheter-site complications, and decreased platelet counts.[71] Based on limited data, heparin therapy may be indicated in as a prophylactic measure in horses with severe sepsis.

Nutritional support improves outcomes in critically ill humans and small animal patients. Horses with acute colitis or typhlocolitis are often partially or completely anorexic as a result of ileus, dysmotility, hypoperfusion, and the systemic inflammatory response. A low-bulk diet, such as a complete pelleted feed, good-quality grass hay, or alfalfa, is recommended for horses with acute colitis.[72] Offering fresh grass may stimulate the appetites of anorectic horses, although large amounts of grass may contribute to the development of laminitis or colic signs. Parenteral nutrition is beneficial in severely catabolic cases of acute colitis that do not tolerate enteral feeding. Parenteral nutrition is indicated in diarrheic patients with anorexia persisting more than 48 to 72 hours and in pregnant and lactating mares.

SUMMARY

The cause of acute, infectious, diarrhea in adult horses is often difficult to define. However, aims of therapy are universal and prompt intervention decreases morbidity and mortality. Furthermore, strong evidence to support many common therapeutic options is lacking, and this should be considered when constructing treatment plans.

REFERENCES

1. Sanchez LC. Pathophysiology of Diarrhea. In: Reed SM, Bayly WM, Sellon DC, editors. Equine internal medicine. vol. 3rd edition. St. Louis(MO): Saunders; 2010. p. 793–866.
2. Cohen ND, Woods AW. Characteristics and risk factors for failure of horses with acute diarrhea to survive: 122 cases (1990-1996). J Am Vet Med Assoc 1999; 214(3):382–90.
3. Belgrave RL, Dickey MM, Arheart KL, et al. Assessment of serum amyloid A testing of horses and its clinical application in a specialized equine practice. J Am Vet Med Assoc 2013;243(1):113–9.
4. Staempfli HR, Townsend HGG, Prescott JF. Prognostic features and clinical presentation of acute idiopathic enterocolitis in horses. Can Vet J 1991;32(2):232–7.
5. Hashimoto-Hill S, Magdesian KG, Kass PH. Serial measurement of lactate concentration in horses with acute colitis. J Vet Intern Med 2011;25(6):1414–9.
6. Weese JS, Baird JD, Poppe C, et al. Emergence of Salmonella typhimurium definitive type 104 (DT104) as an important cause of salmonellosis in horses in Ontario. Can Vet J 2001;42(10):788–92.

7. Kurowski B, Traub-dargatz JL, Morley PS, et al. Detection of *Salmonella* spp in fecal specimens by use of real-time polymerase chain reaction assay. Am J Vet Res 2002;63(9):1256–68.

8. Timoney J. Salmonella infections in horses. In: Barrow PA, Methner U, editors. Salmonella in domestic animals. 2nd edition. Oxfordshire(UK): CABI; 2013. p. 305–17.

9. Ekiri AB, MacKay RJ, Gaskin JM, et al. Epidemiologic analysis of nosocomial salmonella infections in hospitalized horses. J Am Vet Med Assoc 2009;234(1): 108–19.

10. Ernst NS, Hernandez JA, MacKay RJ, et al. Risk factors associated with fecal salmonella shedding among hospitalized horses with signs of gastrointestinal tract disease. J Am Vet Med Assoc 2004;225(2):275–81.

11. Alinovi CA, Ward MP, Couëtil LL, et al. Risk factors for fecal shedding of *Salmonella* from horses in a veterinary teaching hospital. Prev Vet Med 2003;60(4): 307–17.

12. Cohen ND, Martin LJ, Simpson RB, et al. Comparison of polymerase chain reaction and microbiological culture for detection of salmonellae in equine feces and environmental samples. Am J Vet Res 1996;57(6):780–6.

13. Schoster A, Arroyo LG, Staempfli HR, et al. Presence and molecular characterization of *Clostridium difficile* and *Clostridium perfringens* in intestinal compartments of healthy horses. BMC Vet Res 2012;8(94):1–6.

14. Schoster A, Staempfli H. Epidemiology and antimicrobial resistance in *Clostridium difficile* with special reference to the horse. Curr Clin Microbiol Rep 2016;3(1):32–41.

15. Magdesian KG, Dujowich M, Madigan JE, et al. Molecular characterization of *Clostridium difficile* isolates from horses in an intensive care unit and association of disease severity with strain type. J Am Vet Med Assoc 2006;228(5):751–5.

16. Magdesian KG, Leutenegger CM. Real-time PCR and typing of *Clostridium difficile* isolates colonizing mare-foal pairs. Vet J 2011;190(1):119–23.

17. Elmer GW, McFarland LV. Biotherapeutic agents in the treatment of infectious diarrhea. Gastroenterol Clin North Am 2001;30(3):837–54.

18. van Nood E, Vrieze A, Nieuwdorp M, et al. Duodenal infusion of donor feces for recurrent *Clostridium difficile*. N Engl J Med 2013;368(5):407–15.

19. Mullen KR, Yasuda K, Divers TJ, et al. Equine faecal microbiota transplant: current knowledge, proposed guidelines and future directions. Equine Vet Educ 2016;1–10.

20. Waters M, Raju D, Garmory HS, et al. Regulated expression of the beta2-toxin gene (cpb2) in *Clostridium perfringens* type A isolates from horses with gastrointestinal diseases. J Clin Microbiol 2005;43(8):4002–9.

21. Gohari IM, Arroyo L, MacInnes JI, et al. Characterization of *Clostridium perfringens* in the feces of adult horses and foals with acute enterocolitis. Can J Vet Res 2014;78(1):1–7.

22. Lawler JB, Hassel DM, Magnuson RJ, et al. Absorptive effects of di-tri-octahedral smectite on *Clostridium perfringens* alpha, beta, and beta-2 exotoxins and equine colostral antibodies. Am J Vet Res 2008;69(2):233–9.

23. Weese JS, Cote NM, deGannes RVG. Evaluation of in vitro properties of di-tri-octahedral smectite on clostridial toxins and growth. Equine Vet J 2003;35(7): 638–41.

24. Oue Y, Ishihara R, Edamatsu H, et al. Isolation of an equine coronavirus from adult horses with pyrogenic and enteric disease and its antigenic and genomic

characterization in comparison with the NC99 strain. Vet Microbiol 2011;150: 41–8.

25. Pusterla N, Mapes S, Wademan C, et al. Emerging outbreaks associated with equine coronavirus in adult horses. Vet Microbiol 2013;162(1):228–31.

26. Giannitti F, Diab S, Mete A, et al. Necrotizing enteritis and hyperammonemic encephalopathy associated with equine coronavirus infection in equids. Vet Pathol 2015;52(6):1148–56.

27. Xiong Q, Bekebrede H, Sharma P, et al. An ecotype of *Neorickettsia risticii* causing Potomac horse fever in Canada. Appl Environ Microbiol 2016;82(19): 6030–6.

28. Pusterla N, Johnson EM, Chae JS, et al. Digenetic trematodes, *Acanthatrium* sp. and *Lecithodendrium* sp., as vectors of *Neorickettsia risticii*, the agent of Potomac horse fever. J Helminthol 2003;77(4):335–9.

29. Mott J, Muramatsu Y, Seaton E, et al. Molecular analysis of *Neorickettsia risticii* in adult aquatic insects in Pennsylvania, in horses infected by ingestion of insects, and isolated in cell culture. J Clin Microbiol 2002;40(2):690–3.

30. Bertin FR, Reising A, Slovis NM, et al. Clinical and clinicopathological factors associated with survival in 44 horses with equine neorickettsiosis (Potomac horse fever). J Vet Intern Med 2013;27(6):1528–34.

31. Madigan JE, Rikihisa Y, Palmer JE, et al. Evidence for a high rate of false-positive results with the indirect fluorescent antibody test for *Ehrlichia risticii* antibody in horses. J Am Vet Med Assoc 1995;207(11):1448–53.

32. Mott J, Rikihisa Y, Zhang Y, et al. Comparison of PCR and culture to the indirect fluorescent-antibody test for diagnosis of Potomac horse fever. J Clin Microbiol 1997;35(9):2215–9.

33. Atwill ER, Mohammed HO. Evaluation of vaccination of horses as a strategy to control equine monocytic ehrlichiosis. J Am Vet Med Assoc 1996;208(8):1290–4.

34. Dutta SK, Vemulapalli R, Biswas B. Association of deficiency in antibody response to vaccine and heterogeneity of *Ehrlichia risticii* strains with Potomac horse fever vaccine failure in horses. J Clin Microbiol 1998;36(2):506–12.

35. Seahorn JL, Seahorn TL. Fluid therapy in horses with gastrointestinal disease. Vet Clin North Am Equine Pract 2003;19(3):665–79.

36. Jones PA, Tomasic M, Gentry PA. Oncotic, hemodilutional, and hemostatic effects of isotonic saline and hydroxyethyl starch solutions in clinically normal ponies. Am J Vet Res 1997;58(5):541–8.

37. Jones PA, Bain FT, Byars TD, et al. Effect of hydroxyethyl starch infusion on colloid oncotic pressure in hypoproteinemic horses. J Am Vet Med Assoc 2001;218(7):1130–5.

38. Bellezzo F, Kuhnmuench T, Hackett ES. The effect of colloid formulation on colloid osmotic pressure in horses with naturally occurring gastrointestinal disease. BMC Vet Res 2014;10(Suppl S8):1–5.

39. Pantaleon LG, Furr MO, McKenzie HC, et al. Cardiovascular and pulmonary effects of hetastarch plus hypertonic saline solutions during experimental endotoxemia in anesthetized horses. J Vet Intern Med 2006;20(6):1422–8.

40. Pantaleon LG, Furr MO, McKenzie HC, et al. Effects of small- and large-volume resuscitation on coagulation and electrolytes during experimental endotoxemia in anesthetized horses. J Vet Intern Med 2007;21(6):1374–9.

41. Blong AE, Epstein KL, Brainard BM. In vitro effects of three formulations of hydroxyethyl starch solutions on coagulation and platelet function in horses. Am J Vet Res 2013;74(5):712–20.

42. Epstein KL, Bergren A, Giguère S, et al. Cardiovascular, colloid osmotic pressure, and hemostatic effects of 2 formulations of hydroxyethyl starch in healthy horses. J Vet Intern Med 2014;28(1):223–33.

43. Dellinger RP, Levy MM, Rhodes A, et al. Surviving sepsis campaign: International guidelines for management of severe sepsis and septic shock, 2012. Intensive Care Med 2013;39(2):165–228.

44. McKenzie EC, Esser MM, McNitt SE, et al. Effect of infusion of equine plasma or 6% hydroxyethyl starch (600/0.75) solution on plasma colloid osmotic pressure in healthy horses. Am J Vet Res 2016;77(7):708–14.

45. Grønvold AMR, L'Abée-Lund TM, Strand E, et al. Fecal microbiota of horses in the clinical setting: potential effects of penicillin and general anesthesia. Vet Microbiol 2010;145(3–4):366–72.

46. Costa MC, Stämpfli HR, Arroyo LG, et al. Changes in the equine fecal microbiota associated with the use of systemic antimicrobial drugs. BMC Vet Res 2015; 11(19):1–12.

47. Costa MC, Arroyo LG, Allen-Vercoe E, et al. Comparison of the fecal microbiota of healthy horses and horses with colitis by high throughput sequencing of the V3-V5 region of the 16s rRNA gene. PLoS One 2012;7(7):1–12.

48. House JK, Mainar-Jaime RC, Smith BP, et al. Risk factors for nosocomial salmonella infection among hospitalized horses. J Am Vet Med Assoc 1999;214(10): 1511–6.

49. Moore JN, Barton MH. Treatment of endotoxemia. Vet Clin North Am Equine Pract 2003;19(3):681–95.

50. Jackman BR, Moore JN, Barton MH, et al. Comparison of the effects of ketoprofen and flunixin meglumine on the in vitro response of equine peripheral blood monocytes to bacterial endotoxin. Can J Vet Res 1994;58(2):138–43.

51. Semrad SD, Hardee GE, Hardee MM, et al. Low dose flunixin meglumine: effects on eicosanoid production and clinical signs induced by experimental endotoxaemia in horses. Equine Vet J 1987;19(3):201–6.

52. Morresey PR, MacKay RJ. Endotoxin-neutralizing activity of polymyxin B in blood after IV administration in horses. Am J Vet Res 2006;67(4):642–7.

53. Parviainen AK, Barton MH, Norton NN. Evaluation of polymyxin B in an ex vivo of endotoxemia in horses. Am J Vet Res 2001;62(1):72–6.

54. Forbes G, Church S, Savage CJ, et al. Effects of hyperimmune equine plasma on clinical and cellular responses in a low-dose endotoxaemia model in horses. Res Vet Sci 2012;92(1):40–4.

55. Liska DA, Akucewich LH, Marsella R, et al. Pharmacokinetics of pentoxifylline and its 5-hydroxyhexyl metabolite after oral and intravenous administration of pentoxifylline to healthy adult horses. Am J Vet Res 2006;67(9):1621–7.

56. Barton MH, Moore JN, Norton N. Effects of pentoxifylline infusion on response of horses to in vivo challenge exposure with endotoxin. Am J Vet Res 1997;58(11): 1300–7.

57. Baskett A, Barton MH, Norton N, et al. Effect of pentoxifylline, flunixin meglumine, and their combination on a model of endotoxemia in horses. Am J Vet Res 1997; 58(11):1291–9.

58. Edmunds JL, Worgan HJ, Dougal K, et al. In vitro analysis of the effect of supplementation with activated charcoal on the equine hindgut. J Equine Sci 2016; 27(2):49–55.

59. Desrochers AM, Dolente BA, Roy M-F, et al. Efficacy of Saccharomyces boulardii for treatment of horses with acute enterocolitis. J Am Vet Med Assoc 2005;227: 954–9.

60. Boyle AG, Magdesian KG, Durando MM, et al. *Saccharomyces boulardii* viability and efficacy in horses with antimicrobial-induced diarrhoea. Vet Rec 2013;172:128.
61. Schoster A, Staempfli HR, Abrahams M, et al. Effect of a probiotic on prevention of diarrhea and *Clostridium difficile* and *Clostridium perfringens* shedding in foals. J Vet Intern Med 2015;29(3):925–31.
62. Furr M. Orally administered *Pediococcus acidilactici* and *Saccharomyces boulardii*-based probiotics alter select equine immune function parameters. J Equine Vet Sci 2014;34(10):1156–63.
63. Weese JS. Microbiologic evaluation of commercial probiotics. J Am Vet Med Assoc 2002;220(6):794–7.
64. Scott Weese J, Martin H. Assessment of commercial probiotic bacterial contents and label accuracy. Can Vet J 2011;52(1):43–6.
65. Tleyjeh IM, Bin Abdulhak AA, Riaz M, et al. Association between proton pump inhibitor therapy and *Clostridium difficile* infection: a contemporary systematic review and meta-analysis. PLoS One 2012;7:e50836.
66. Furr M, Cohen ND, Axon JE, et al. Treatment with histamine-type 2 receptor antagonists and omeprazole increase the risk of diarrhoea in neonatal foals treated in intensive care units. Equine Vet J 2012;44(Suppl. 41):80–6.
67. Van Eps AW, Pollitt CC. Equine laminitis model: lamellar histopathology seven days after induction with oligofructose. Equine Vet J 2009;41(8):735–40.
68. Divers TJ. Clinical application of current research findings toward the prevention and treatment of acute laminitis in horses with systemic inflammatory diseases: an internist's perspective. J Equine Vet Sci 2010;30(9):517–24.
69. Liu X-L, Want X-Z, Liu X-X, et al. Low-dose heparin as treatment for early disseminated intravascular coagulation during sepsis: a prospective clinical study. Exp Ther Med 2014;7:604–8.
70. De La Rebière Pouyade G, Grulke S, Detilleux J, et al. Evaluation of low-molecular-weight heparin for the prevention of equine laminitis after colic surgery: retrospective study. J Vet Emerg Crit Care (San Antonio) 2009;19(1):113–9.
71. Feige K, Schwarzwald CC, Bombeli T. Comparison of unfractioned and low molecular weight heparin for prophylaxis of coagulopathies in 52 horses with colic: a randomised double-blind clinical trial. Equine Vet J 2003;35(5):506–13.
72. Gary Magdesian K. Nutrition for critical gastrointestinal illness: feeding horses with diarrhea or colic. Vet Clin North Am Equine Pract 2003;19(3):617–44.

Foal Diarrhea
Established and Postulated Causes, Prevention, Diagnostics, and Treatments

Olimpo Oliver-Espinosa, DVM, MSc, DVSc

KEYWORDS

• Foal • Infections • Enterocolitis • Diagnosis • Therapy

KEY POINTS

- Diarrhea is one of the most important diseases in young foals and may occur in more than half of foals until weaning age.
- Several infectious and noninfectious underlying causes have been implicated but scientific evidence of pathogenesis is constantly evolving.
- Practically it is important to investigate all known different potential causes and to identify infectious agents to avoid outbreaks, as well as to evaluate in individuals the level of systemic compromise and establish an adequate therapy.
- In addition it is crucial to differentiate foals that can be managed in field conditions from those who should be sent to a referral center.
- This article reviews these aspects and recent developments in the diagnostic and therapeutic approaches.

INTRODUCTION

Diarrhea is defined as increased frequency of defecation with increased water content in feces.[1] Foals that develop diarrhea usually have enteritis, which is associated with systemic inflammatory response syndrome (SIRS).[2] More than 50% of foals experience 1 or more bouts of diarrhea in the first 6 months of life.[3–5] There are established and putative infectious and noninfectious causes of foal diarrhea. Treatment is mainly symptomatic but some specific treatments of various causes are available.

PATIENT HISTORY

Vaccination and worming status, information on number and ages of the affected foals, and hygienic conditions on the farm are important.[6,7] Failure of passive transfer of immunity might be reported.[8] Diarrhea commonly occurs within the first 6 months of

Department of Animal Health, National University of Colombia, Carrera 45 # 26-85, Edif. Uriel Gutiérrez, Bogotá D.C., Colombia
E-mail address: ojolivere@unal.edu.co

Vet Clin Equine 34 (2018) 55–68
https://doi.org/10.1016/j.cveq.2017.11.003
0749-0739/18/© 2017 Elsevier Inc. All rights reserved.

life. Depending on the etiology, outbreaks can occur, or single foals might be affected.[9,10] Risk factors include suboptimal deworming of mares and extensive use of antibiotics.[4] Additional observations can be depression, decreased suckling reflex, weakness, colic, weight loss, and occasionally sudden death.[8]

CLINICAL PRESENTATION

Clinical signs vary.[6,7] Initial signs may include colic, hypermotility or amotility, and abdominal distension. Fecal consistency can range from watery to pasty, with different colors, and may contain blood or casts.[7] Foals tend to dehydrate quickly and can reach severe dehydration evidenced by sunken eyeballs and a prolonged skin tent. Depression, weakness, anorexia, salivation, and bruxism are frequently observed. Body temperature varies from fever to hypothermia.[2] Cases of enteritis commonly have signs of SIRS, including congested mucous membranes, tachycardia, weak pulses, tachypnea, and cool extremities.[2,7] When signs progress, recumbence, coma, and death may occur.[7] Up to 50% of diarrheic foals less than 30 days of age with diarrhea are bacteremic.[11,12]

CLINICAL PATHOLOGY

If dehydration is present, hematocrit is high.[13] Signs of inflammation are present in the leukogram, including leukopenia or leukocytosis, commonly due to abnormal neutrophil counts. A left shift might also be present, particularly in cases with SIRS.[11] Plasma total proteins can be increased or decreased, as in cases with sepsis, protein-losing inflammation (salmonellosis), or *Lawsonia intracellularis* infections.[14,15] Acute phase proteins, such as fibrinogen and serum amyloid A, are usually elevated.[13]

Electrolyte derangements are common and should be evaluated. Up to 66% of the foals have been reported as hyponatremic and 33% hypokalemic. Hyperchloremia or hypochloremia also can occur.[13] Foals with diarrhea usually have a strong ion metabolic acidosis with low blood pH, low plasma bicarbonate levels, and a decreased strong ion difference (strong ion difference = Na + K-Cl lactate = 36–44) due to electrolyte derangements.[11,13] Increased lactate concentrations are also common and contribute to the low SID.

Urea and creatinine levels are often increased, indicating a prerenal and occasionally also a renal azotemia.[11]

ETIOLOGY

Noninfectious causes include foal heat diarrhea, perinatal asphyxia syndrome, necrotizing enterocolitis (NEC), dietary imbalance, equine gastric ulcer syndrome, luminal irritant diarrhea, and secondary lactose intolerance.[16,17]

The most common infectious agents include rotavirus (RV), *Clostridium perfringens* types A and C, *Salmonella* spp, *C difficile*, *Cryptosporidia*, and *L intracellularis*.[2,3,6,11,15,17] Less common causes are *Coronavirus*, *Rhodococcus equi*, and *Strongyloides westeri*.[18–20] Single case reports have also been published on *Aeromona hydrophyla*,[21] *Neorickettsia risticii*,[22] candida[23] and *Listeria monocytogenes*.[24] Coinfections can occur,[22] as with *C perfringens* and *C difficile*.[25]

Foal Heat Diarrhea

Foal heat diarrhea is usually a self-limiting condition in foals aged 5 days to 15 days. It occurs in 75% to 80% of neonatal foals and usually lasts 3 days to 4 days.[16] These foals have diarrhea, show no signs of systemic disease, and continue to suckle well.[2] Individual foals may be affected by more severe and prolonged diarrheic episodes.[16] The etiology remains speculative and include changes in mare's milk composition during foal heat; however, orphan foals on milk replacer developed diarrhea at similar ages, making this theory less likely.[26] More recently, maturational changes in bacterial intestinal flora during that early life period have been elucidated and this adaptation of the microbiota may lead to foal heat diarrhea.[27]

Rotavirus

RVs are currently the most frequently detected infectious agents in foals with diarrhea.[11,22] In a study using real-time polymerase chain reaction (PCR), RV was responsible for 35% to 90% of cases up to 3 months of age.[11] RV belongs to the Reoviridae, subfamily Sedoreovirinae, genus *Rotavirus*. Only group A has been associated with horse infection.[28,29] RVs tend to cause outbreaks, have an ubiquitous world distribution in the horse population, are highly contagious, replicate rapidly, and are shed in high concentrations in feces of affected animals.[2,30] Transmission is via the feco-oral route of contaminated feces or fomites. The incubation period is 1 day to 4 days.[28] Virus shedding can start before the onset of diarrhea, persists during the clinical phase, and may persist for up to12 days post resolution of diarrhea.[31] Foals with RV diarrhea presented to a referral hospital had a survival rate of 94%.[11]

RV diarrhea is primarily malabsorptive but also includes a toxin-mediated secretory component.[32] It preferentially infects the mature absorptive villous enterocytes of duodenum, jejunum, and ileum-sparing crypts, causing villous damage resulting in malabsorptive diarrhea.[32] Foals often become lactose intolerant because lactase is mainly produced by the brush border epithelium of the villous enterocyte. The RV nonstructural glycoprotein 4 (NSP4) is a viral enterotoxin, responsible for the hypersecretory component of RV diarrhea.[33]

Clostridium perfringens

C perfringens is a gram-positive anaerobic spore-forming bacterium, associated with enterocolitis in foals and horses.[30,34] *C perfringens* was long considered part of normal microbiota of the large colon, but recent studies found low prevalence (0%–8%) in feces of horses.[35,36] In neonatal foals *C perfringens* was isolated from the feces of 90% of 3-day-old foals but isolation rates decreased over the first weeks of life.[37] The most common genotype identified (85%) is type A; *C perfringens* type C was isolated in less than 1% to 3% of neonatal foals.[37,38] In a retrospective study, *C perfringens* was the second most significant organism isolated from foals with diarrhea.[11] In some instances, *C perfringens* may cause sudden death without prior clinical manifestations. Foal diarrhea associated with *C perfringens* occurs commonly early in life; 96% of affected foals had adequate transfer of passive immunity.[34] Diarrheic foals less than 1 month of age were significantly more likely to be positive for *C perfringens* (odds ratio [OR] 15; 95% CI, 3.5–66) compared with older foals.[11] Reported mortality rates vary from 12% to 83%.[11,22] The highest mortality has been reported for infection with *C perfringens* type C.[34]

C perfringens type A produces α toxin; type B produces α, β, and ε toxins; type C produces α and β toxins; type D produces α and ε toxins; and type E produces α and ι toxins.[35] Additional virulence factors include β2 toxin,[39] an enterotoxin produced by all *C perfringens* but most commonly by type A.[2,35] Recently, an additional toxin named *netF* has been identified in foals with NEC and in vitro cell cytotoxicity has been proved.[40] The role of these additional virulence factors in pathogenesis of diarrhea is still debated.

Salmonellosis

Salmonella spp are rod-shaped, gram-negative Enterobacteriaceae.[41] There are currently more than 2200 serovars in 8 subspecies, with subspecies I responsible for 99% of clinical mammalian diseases.[41] The most frequent *Salmonella* serovars isolated from horses in the United States include Typhimurium, Newport, Anatum, Javiana, and Agona.[41] Transmission mainly occurs via the feco-oral route.[42] Diarrheic foals older than 1 month of age were significantly more likely to have fecal *Salmonella* isolated than younger foals (OR 2.6; 95% CI, 1.2–6.0).[11]

Salmonella colonizes the intestine using the invasion-associated type III secretion system causing inflammation and massive mucosal damage of the ileum and colon.[42]

Clostridium difficile

C difficile is a gram-positive, anaerobic, spore-forming bacterium commonly associated with diarrhea and colitis in humans and other mammals.[35] It is considered among the most important agents of enteric disease of foals and adult horses.[11,17] *C difficile* enterocolitis in foals has been reproduced experimentally.[43] *C difficile* has been isolated from healthy and diarrheic foals and adult horses.[44] Carrier rates in healthy foals are higher at 2 weeks of age compared with older foals.[38] It has been isolated in 11% of diarrheic foals.[38] There have been limited studies on risk factors, but antibiotic administration and hospitalization seem the most important ones.[44] Transmission occurs via fecal oral route.

The 2 major toxins, toxin A (TcdA) an enterotoxin and toxin B (TcdB) a cytotoxin,[45] are responsible for causing increased paracellular permeability of mucosal surfaces, cell rounding, and eventually cell death or apoptosis.[45] The toxins also cause inflammation resulting in increased fluid exudation and mucosal damage, leading to diarrhea or pseudomembranous colitis.[45]

Less Common Infectious and Parasitic Agents

Coronavirus

Equine coronavirus is considered an enteropathogen in foals.[11,18] The prevalence rates of equine coronavirus in healthy and diarrheic foals in central Kentucky were 27% and 29%, respectively.[22] The importance of this agent is not known.

Cryptosporidium

Cryptosporidium spp can infect adult horses and foals, *Crystosporidium parvum* is the most common genotype identified.[46] Infection occurs with ingested oocysts that reach the ileum. It affects mainly foals with severe combined immunodeficiency (SCID), but outbreaks in immune-competent foals have also been reported.[47] Self-limiting diarrhea can occur for up to 8 days and in older foals; chronic and intermittent diarrhea may also occur.[46]

Lawsonia intracellularis

L intracellularis is a gram-negative obligate intracellular bacterium affecting mainly foals aged 4 months to 7 months (range 2–13 months) causing proliferative enteropathy.[48] In 2 recent studies using fecal PCR in healthy and diarrheic foals, it was not found in foals less than 4 month of age.[11,22] It is transmitted via the feco-oral route.[48]

Rhodococcus equi

R equi, a gram-positive facultative intracellular pathogen, is a common etiologic agent in foal pneumonia.[49] It has been reported that up to 50% of foals with *R equi* bronchopneumonia also had intestinal lesions on necropsy, and 4% of foals had intestinal lesions without pneumonia.[49]

Sepsis in foals

Diarrhea is common in septic foals, due to hemodynamic alterations leading to gastro-intestinal (GI) mucosal hypoperfusion, inflammatory mediators associated with SIRS, and dysmotility.[2]

Other Infectious Agents

The role of enterotoxigenic *Escherichia coli* in foal diarrhea has been suggested, but there is only 1 report of a single case where it was proposed as causative agent.[50] *Aeromona aerophila* has been isolated from 9% of diarrheic foals[51] but its role in foal diarrhea is unknown. *S westeri* infects foals early in its life, but its role in diarrhea is questionable; however, in 1 study it was associated with diarrhea when fecal egg count was greater than 2000 eggs/g of feces.[20] Enterotoxigenic *Bacteroides fragilis* was isolated from the feces of 10 of 40 Thoroughbred foals with naturally acquired diarrhea.[52] In another study, using PCR, *N risticii* was found in 4% of foals with diarrhea.[22] The importance of the latter 2 agents is currently unknown.

NONINFECTIOUS DIARRHEA

Necrotizing Enterocolitis

NEC is a disease primarily of premature infants and consists of necrotic injury to the mucosal and submucosal layers of the GI tract. The distal small intestine and proximal colon are most commonly affected.[2] NEC has been reported in foals. These foals showed severe weakness, inability to stand, colic, ileus, gastric reflux, intolerance to enteral feeding, shock signs, and evidence of pneumatosis intestinalis in the large colon.[53]

Hypoxic Gastrointestinal Damage

Peripartum asphyxia syndrome in foals can cause ischemic damage to different organs, such as GI tract, kidneys, heart, and brain.[54]

Equine Gastric Ulcer Syndrome and Diarrhea

Equine gastric ulcer syndrome occurs in foals from 2 days to 9 months of age[17] and has been associated with diarrhea; however, a recent consensus statement questions this association.[55]

Luminal Irritant Diarrhea

Foals can develop pica and may ingest large amounts of sand or other abrasive materials that can be extremely irritating and damaging to intestinal mucosa that may result in diarrhea with colic.[17]

Diarrhea Due To Lactose Intolerance

Primary lactose intolerance in foals is rare.[56] Secondary lactose intolerance produced by small intestinal enteritis associated with RV and *C difficile* has been also reported.[57,58]

Dietary Diarrhea

Dietary intolerance in foals can cause diarrhea. It is more commonly seen in foals receiving enteral nutrition with milk replacers.[2,17]

DIAGNOSIS

Establishing a diagnosis of diarrhea is easily achieved whereas establishing the cause of the diarrhea is often difficult. The minimum database of a foal with diarrhea should include a thorough history, physical examination, complete blood cell count, biochemistry profile, and determination of serum immunoglobulin concentrations. If available or in severe cases, blood gas analysis can also be useful. Abdominal ultrasound can be useful to determine signs of NEC and to assess intestinal wall thickness. Abdominal radiography can be used to determine presence of sand and gas accumulations. A major differential in diarrheic foals is sepsis and if available a sepsis score and blood culture should be performed.

Additionally, fecal testing is recommended and tests should be based on the most likely causative agent of a given case based on age and clinical signs (**Table 1**). Testing options for various causes are presented in **Table 2**. Fecal panels are offered by various laboratories, but results have to be interpreted with caution, because they have not been critically validated. A positive diagnostic test does not always confirm that this agent is the etiologic cause of the diarrhea. Several pathogens can be found in feces of healthy as well as diarrheic animals.

INITIAL RESUSCITATION
Rehydration

To correct hypovolemia, crystalloids, colloids, or combinations of these 2 can be used. Replacement crystalloid fluids for foals include lactated Ringer solution, Normosol R, and Plasma-Lyte 148.[59] Hypertonic solutions are not commonly used in foals, because foals may not be tolerant of large sodium loads.[60] Synthetic colloids can be used as 3-mL/kg to 5-mL/kg boluses if needed.[60] Synthetic colloids have been associated with renal failure and a worse outcome in human medicine and their use is currently questioned in horses as well. An attempt should be made to correct hypovolemia without synthetic colloids if deemed feasible. Plasma is in foals a better choice of colloids than synthetic colloids. In case colloids are used, administration as constant rate infusion (CRI) of 1 mL/kg/h to 2 mL/kg/h to has been suggested to avoid or minimize the risks for anaphylactoid reactions.[60]

Table 1	
Common infectious agents of foal diarrhea sorted by age range of foals	
Age Range	**Common Causes**
< Two weeks	Foal heat diarrhea
	C perfringens
	Rotavirus
	C difficile
	Septicemia
	Cryptosporidium
	Neonatal asphyxia
	NCE
Two weeks–two months	Rotavirus
	Cryptosporidium
	Salmonella spp
	S westeri
> Two mo	L intracellularis
	S westeri
	N risticii
All ages	Salmonella spp
	Lactose intolerance
	Luminal irritants

Table 2
Diagnostic tests for associated causes of foal diarrhea

Etiologic Agent	Test	Characteristics
Foal heat diarrhea	Clinical examination	Based on clinical presentation
RV	Electron microscopy	Limited use in the field
	Latex particle agglutination	Sensitivity not as high as ELISA, rapid, simple, and useful in the field
	ELISA	Most show high sensitivity
	RT-PCR	Commercially available, rapid and sensitive
C perfringens	Fecal culture	Considered normal GI inhabitant in horses, but recent studies have not confirmed it.
	PCR	Detect toxin genes, best suited as adjunctive test because toxigenic strains are often found in healthy horses.
	ELISA	To detect specific toxins, it is deemed more accurate than gene detection PCR
	ELISA + toxin gene PCR	The strongest evidence of C perfringens–associated disease
Salmonella	Fecal culture	Isolation is criterium of diagnosis; 5 daily consecutive samplings in adult horses have 97% sensitivity. Number of samples not determined in foals.
	PCR	Sensitivity from 80% to 100% and specificity that ranged from 85% to 98%. Potential for misclassification
C difficile	Fecal culture	Isolation is not confirmatory. Normal horses may harbor it, and there are nontoxigenic strains
	CTA	Best available test, but technically demanding, time consuming, and not readily available
	PCR for TcdA and TcdB	High sensitivity, short turnaround time. False positives in carriers
	Toxin A/B ELISA,	Some tests validated in horses. Reported sensitivity and specificity of 84% and 96%, respectively, compared with CTA
Coronavirus	RT-PCR	High sensitivity. There are other tests such virus isolation, immunofluorescent antibody test, virus neutralization. Significance of detection not determined yet.
Cryptosporidium	Fecal modified AF	Low cost and simple methodology but low sensitivity
	PCR	High sensitivity and specificity
	ELISA	Similar sensitivity to AF
L intracellularis	PCR	Indicates bacteria shedding and active infection
	Warthin-Steiner silver stain	Postmortem diagnosis. Strongly suggestive. The curved bacilli presence
R equi	PCR	Has been used in foals with diarrhea
S westeri	Fecal flotation	Commonly used
Lactose intolerance	Intestinal lactose absorption test	Commonly used to determine it

Abbreviations: AF, acid-fast stain; CTA, cell cytotoxicity assay; RT-PCR, reverse transcription–PCR.

The speed and volume of infusions depend on the degree of hypovolemic, cardiovascular status and plasma protein levels; however, there are no studies in foals to suggest accurate fluid rates. The most recent recommendation based on pediatric patients suggests an initial fluid bolus of 20 mL/kg crystalloid solution over 10 minutes to 20 minutes.[59] Perfusion should be reassessed after the bolus and, if still inadequate, this bolus can be repeated up to 3 times in total. Clinical signs of adequate perfusion include normalization of tachycardia, improvement in mentation, return of suckle reflex, and urine voidance. If possible, laboratory parameters should be reevaluated. After 3 boluses, continuous rate infusion of fluids is recommended if possible. If response to fluid therapy is inadequate (perfusion does not normalize), inotrope therapy should be added. Dobutamine diluted in isotonic saline, 5% dextrose, or lactated Ringer solution is used and the dose should be titrated from 1 µg/kg/min to 3 µg/kg/min up to 5 µg/kg/min CRI. The remainder of the dehydration should be corrected in within 12 hours to 24 hours and ongoing losses added to the fluid regimen.

Maintenance

Maintenance amounts of fluid need to be added if the foal is not allowed to nurse. The maintenance fluid needs in foals should be calculated using the Holliday-Segar formula for body weight (BW)[59]:

1 kg to 10 kg = 100 mL/kg/d

11 kg to 20 kg = 1000 mL + 50 mL for each kg >10 kg/d

Greater than 20 kg of weight = 1500 mL+25 mL for each kg/d >20 kg

Correction of electrolyte imbalances during maintenance fluid therapy is crucial for recovery. This also aids in balancing the acid base status of foals. Hyponatremia should be corrected at a rate not exceeding 0.5 mEq/h to avoid central pontine myelinolysis. Hyponatremia can be partially corrected by increasing the plasma sodium concentration by 2 mEq/L to 4 mEq/L to abolish seizure activity.[60] Hypokalemia is treated with empiric supplementation of fluids with 10 mEq/L to 40 mEq/L of potassium chloride and it depends on the existing plasma potassium concentration. Hyperkalemia can be empirically treated with administration of 20 mL/kg of 0.9% sodium chloride containing calcium (eg, 0.4 mEq/L to 1 mL/kg of 23% calcium borogluconate) and 4 mg/kg/min to 8 mg/kg/min of dextrose.[60] Isotonic sodium bicarbonate (1.3%) can be used with added dextrose as an alternative treatment. In refractory and severe cases of hyperkalemia, insulin treatment can be tried.

Sodium bicarbonate therapy should be reserved for foals with severe refractory acidosis, often due to hyperchloremia. In these cases, isotonic sodium bicarbonate (1.3%) intravenously (IV) can help ameliorate signs of acidosis by supplying sodium while decreasing the chloride load. Alternatively oral sodium bicarbonate can be administered.

All foals with compromised systemic status usually benefit from glucose administration. A starting dose is 4 mg/kg/min. The rate can be increased to 6 mg/kg/min to 8 mg/kg/min if needed.[60,61] Glucose should be administered separately from fluid therapy if possible, using a fluid pump. This allows adjusting fluid and glucose therapy separately.

ANTI-INFLAMMATORY AND ANTIENDOTOXIC TREATMENTS

Nonsteroidal anti-inflammatory drugs (NSAIDs) should be used cautiously in foals less than 1 month old due to renal and gastric side effects.[2] Polymyxin B (6000 U/kg IV) can be used to treat endotoxemia.[62] Plasma transfusion should be considered for foals with failure of passive transfer of immunity. Because foals with diarrhea may use their globulins despite initially adequate levels, assessment of immunoglobulin concentration should be repeated periodically to assess the need for further plasma transfusion.

Absorptive Agents

Adsorptive agents, such as kaolin/pectin and bismuth subsalicylate, have been used but efficacy studies are lacking. These agents are used at 0.5 mL/kg to 4 mL/kg, 1 to 4 times daily.[63]

Di-tri-octahedral smectite can has been shown to neutralize C difficile and C perfringens toxins in vitro. It is possible that in vivo neutralization of bacterial toxins in the gut could also occur.[64]

Modification of the Gastrointestinal Microbiota

The use of probiotics in neonatal foals cannot be recommended based on currently available data. The use of fecal microbiota transplant has been proposed based on its remarkable success in treating recurrent C difficile infection in humans[65] (see Marcio Carvalho Costa and Jeffery Scott Weese's article, "Understanding the Intestinal Microbiome in Health and Disease," in this issue).

Adjunct Therapies

The prophylactic use of antiulcer medications is controversial in neonatal foals but indicated in older foals. It has been shown that neonatal foals on antiulcer medication had a higher risk of developing diarrhea.[66] Omeprazole is the only approved drug for the treatment of EGUS, and 4 mg/kg orally, every 24 hours, is the recommended dose.[49]

Gastroprotectants should be considered if NSAIDs are given for prolonged periods of time.

In foals with signs of SIRS or sepsis, the use of broad-spectrum antibiotics is warranted. The antibiotics commonly used are a combination of aminoglycosides (mainly amikacin 20–25 mg/kg IV every 24 h) and penicillin (22.000–44.000 IU/kg IV every 6 h).[67]

Specific Therapies

Metronidazole (15–25 mg/kg body weight every 8 h) is widely used for clostridial diarrhea, but there are no current objective data supporting its use.[67] Vancomycin has been used in cases of resistance and in humans is used in severe cases of C difficile–associated diarrhea.[68–74] Bacitracin was used in the past but is no longer available.[68]

Antibiotic treatment in foals with known Salmonella infection is indicated due to the risk for bacteremia and sepsis. The treatment should be continued beyond clinical recovery to prevent secondary seeding.[6] Antimicrobials effective against Salmonella spp include extended-spectrum cephalosporin or ampicillin-sulbactam alone or in combination with an aminoglycoside (gentamicin or amikacin) or fluorquinolones.[67]

Antimicrobial choices recommended for treating L intracellularis include oxytetracyclines, macrolides, or chloramphenicol.[48] Treatment of rhodococcal enterocolitis is similar to pulmonary R equi infection using macrolide antimicrobials combined with rifampin.[49] Therapy for cryptosporidiosis is largely supportive in foals, but therapy with the aminoglycoside paromomycin could be attempted.[6] In cases of *S westeri*–associated diarrhea, anthelmintics (oxibendazole [15 mg/kg] or ivermectin [0.2 mg/kg]) should be used.[75]

NUTRITIONAL SUPPORT

Foals with mild to moderate diarrhea without evidence of colic should be allowed to continue nursing. In contrast, any foal with abdominal discomfort will likely benefit from a period of brief GI rest (12–24 h).[2] Fluid therapy has to be administered if a foal less than 4 weeks old is not nursing for more than 6 hours. In cases of suspected lactose intolerance, exogenous lactase (Lactaid, 3000–6000 FCC U orally every 6 h) can be used.[2] Reintroduction to feeding should be slow and gradual. Feeding of 10% of body weight per day divided into hourly or 2-hour feeding intervals through a nasogastric tube or feeding tube is an adequate starting level.[76]

PREVENTION AND MANAGEMENT

Foal infectious diarrhea prevention should focus on 3 important aspects of disease prophylaxis: minimize exposure to pathogens (disinfection and isolation), increasing immunity (vaccination), and optimization of management practices.[77]

Detection of a sick foal demands that in-contact animals should not be moved to other locations, because they may be a source of infection. People traffic should be curtailed by ensuring that healthy animals are attended to first, followed by in-contact foals, and finally clinical cases.[78]

REFERENCES

1. Constable P, Hinchcliff KW, Donne SH, et al. Veterinary medicine. 11th edition. St Louis (MO): Elsevier; 2017. p. 175–435.
2. Magdesian KG. Neonatal foal diarrhea. Vet Clin Equine 2005;21:295–312.
3. Traub-Dargaztz JL, Gay CC, Evermann JF, Ward AC, et al. Epidemiological survey of diarrhea in foals. J Am Vet Med Assoc 1988;192:1553–6.
4. Cohen ND. Causes of and farm management factors associated with disease and death in foals. J Am Vet Med Assoc 1994;204:1644–51.
5. Franco MS, Oliver Espinosa OJ. Estudio de la morbilidad, mortalidad y de enfermedades en potros de caballo criollo colombiano durante los 30 primeros dias de vida en la sabana de Bogota. Rev Med Vet 2015;30:67–82.
6. Lester GD. Foal diarrhea. In: Robinson NE, editor. Current therapy in equine medicine. 5th edition. Philadelphia: WB Saunders; 2003. p. 677–80.
7. Knotttenbelt DC, Holdstock N, Madigan JE. Equine neonatology medicine and surgery. Edimburgh (United Kingdom): Saunders; 2004. p. 219–23.
8. Magdesian G. Diarrhea. In: Paradis MR, editor. Equine neonatal medicine : a case base approach. Philadelphia: Elsevier Saundres; 2006. p. 213–21.
9. Wohlfender FD, Barrelet FE, Doherr MG, et al. Diseases in neonatal foals. Part 2: potential risk factors for a higher incidence of infectious diseases during the first 30 days post partum. Equine Vet J 2009;41(2):179–85.
10. Urquhart K. Diarrhoea in foals. In Pract 1981;3:22–3.
11. Frederick J, Giguère S, Sanchez LC. Infectious agents detected in the feces of diarrheic foals: a retrospective study of 233 cases (2003-2008). J Vet Intern Med 2009;23:1254–60.

12. Hollis AR, Wilkins PA, Palmer JE, et al. Bacteremia in equine neonatal diarrhea: a retrospective study (1990-2007). J Vet Intern Med 2008;22:1203-9.

13. Olivo G, Lukas TM, Borges AS, et al. Enteropathogens and coinfections in foals with and without diarrhea. Biomed Res Int 2016;1-12.

14. House JK, Smith BP. Salmonella in horses. In: Wray C, Wray W, editors. Salmonella in domestic animals. New York: CABI Publishing; 2000. p. 219-30.

15. Frazer ML. Lawsonia intracellularis infection in horses: 2005-2007. J Vet Intern Med 2008;22:1243-8.

16. Masri MD, Merritt AM, Gronwall R, et al. Faecal composition in foal heat diarrhea. Equine Vet J 1986;18:301-6.

17. Mallicote M, House AM, Sanchez LC. A review of foal diarrhea from birth to weaning. Equine Vet Educ 2012;24:206-14.

18. Davis E, Rush BR, Cox J, et al. Neonatal enterocolitis associated with coronavirus infectionin a foal: a case report. J Vet Diagn Invest 2000;12:153-6.

19. Zink MC, Yager JA, Smart NL. Corynebacterium equi infections in horses, 1958-1984: a review of 131 cases. Can Vet J 1986;27:213.

20. Netherwood T, Wood JL, Townsend HG, et al. Foal diarrhea between 1991 and 1994 in the United Kingdom associated with Clostridium perfringens, rotavirus, Strongyloides westeri and Cryptosporidium spp. Epidemiol Infect 1996;117:375-83.

21. Browning GF, Chalmers RM, Snodgrass DR, et al. The prevalence of enteric pathogens in diarrhoeic thoroughbred foals in Britain and Ireland. Equine Vet J 1991;23:405-9.

22. Slovis NM, Elam J, Estrada M, et al. Infectious agents associated with diarrhoea in neonatal foals in central Kentucky: a comprehensive molecular study. Equine Vet J 2014;46:311-6.

23. De Bruijin CM, Wijnberg. Potential role of candidad species in antibiotic-associated diarrhea in foals. Vet Rec 2004;155:26-8.

24. Warner SL, Boggs J, Lee JK, et al. Clinical, pathological, and genetic characterization of Listeria monocytogenes causing sepsis and necrotizing typhlocolitis and hepatitis in a foal. J Vet Diagn Invest 2012;24:581-6.

25. Uzal FA, Diab SS, Blanchard P, et al. Clostridium perfringens type C and Clostridium difficile co-infection in foals. Vet Microbiol 2012;156:395-402.

26. Johnston R, Kamstra L, Kohler P. Mares' milk composition as related to 'foal heat' scours. J Anim Sci 1970;31:549-53.

27. Kuhl J, Winterhoff N, Wulfa M, et al. Changes in faecal bacteria and metabolic parameters in foals during the first six weeks of life. Vet Microbiol 2011;151:321-8.

28. Bailey KE, Gilkerson JR, Browning GF. Equine rotaviruses—Current understanding and continuing challenges. Vet Microbiol 2013;167:135-44.

29. Pappa H, Matthijnssens J, Martellac V, et al. Global distribution of group A rotavirus strains in horses: a systematic review. Vaccine 2013;31:5627-33.

30. Wierup M. Equine intestinal clostridiosis: an acute disease in horses associated with high intestinal counts of Clostridium perfringes type A. Acta Vet Scand 1977;62:1-182.

31. Magdesian KG. Viral diarrhea. In: Sellon DC, Long MT, editors. Equine infectious diseases. St Louis (MO): Elsevier; 2014. p. 198-203.

32. Desselberger U. Rotaviruses. Virus Res 2014;190:75-96.

33. Zhang M, Zeng CQ, Morris AP, et al. A functional NSP4 enterotoxin peptide secreted from rotavirus-infected cells. J Virol 2000;74:11663-70.

34. East LM, Savage CJ, Traub-Dargatz JL, et al. Enterocolitis associated with clostridium perfringes infection in neonatal foals : 54 cases (1988-1997). J Am Vet Med Assoc 1998;11:1751–6.

35. Songer JG. Clostridial enteric diseases of domestic animals. Clin Microbiol Rev 1996;9:216–34.

36. Schoster A, Arroyo LG, Staempfli HR, et al. Presence and molecular characterization of Clostridium difficile and Clostridium perfringens in intestinal compartments of healthy horses. BMC Vet Res 2012;8:94–9.

37. Tillotson K, Traub-Dargatz JL, Dickinson CE, et al. Population-based study of fecal shedding of Clostridium perfringens in broodmares and foals. J Am Vet Med Assoc 2002;220(3):342–8.

38. Schoster A, Staempfli HR, Abrahams M, et al. Effect of a probiotic on prevention of diarrhea and clostridium difficile and clostridium perfringens shedding in foals. J Vet Intern Med 2015;29:925–31.

39. Hazlett MJ, Kircanski J, Slavic D, et al. Beta-2 toxigenic Clostridium perfringens type A colitis in a three-day-old foal. J Vet Diagn Invest 2011;23:373–6.

40. Gohari IM, Parreira VM, Nowel VJ, et al. A Novel pore-forming toxin in type A Clostridium perfringens is associated with both fatal canine hemorrhagic gastroenteritis and fatal foal necrotizing enterocolitis. PLoS One 2015;10(4):e0122684.

41. Hernandez JA, Maureen T, Long MT, et al. Salmonelosis. In: Sellon DC, Long MT, editors. Equine infectious diseases. 2nd edition. St Louis (MO): Saunders Elsevier; 2014. p. 322–33.

42. Wray C, Davies R. Salmonella infections in cattle. In: Wray C, Wray W, editors. Salmonella in domestic animals. New York: CABI Publishing; 2000. p. 169–90.

43. Arroyo LG, Keel JS, Staempfli HR. Experimental clostridium difficile enterocolitis in foals. J Vet Intern Med 2004;18:734–8.

44. Gustafsson A, Baverud V, Gunnarsson A, et al. Study of faecal shedding of Clostridium difficile in horses treated with penicillin. Equine Vet J 2004;36:180–2.

45. Diab SS, Songer G, Uzal FA. Clostridium difficile infection in horses: a review. Vet Microbiol 2013;167:42–9.

46. Xiao L, Herd RP. Review of equine Cryptosporidium infection. Equine Vet J 1994; 26:9–13.

47. Imhasly A, Frey CF, Mathis A, et al. Cryptosporidiosis (C. parvum) in a foal with diarrhea. Schweiz Arch Tierheilkd 2009;151:21–6.

48. Pusterla N, Gebhart CJ, Lavoie JP, et al. Lawsonia intracellularis. In: Sellon DC, Long MT, editors. Equine infectious diseases. 2nd edition. St Louis (MO): Saunders Elsevier; 2014. p. 316–21.

49. Giguère S, Cohen ND, Chaffin MK, et al. Diagnosis, treatment, control, and prevention of infections caused by Rhodococcus equi in foals. J Vet Intern Med 2011;25:1209–20.

50. Holland RE, Sriranganathan N, DuPont L. Isolation of enterotoxigenic Escherichia coli from a foal with diarrhea. J Am Vet Med Assoc 1989;194:389–91.

51. Browning GF, Chalmers RM, Snodgrass DR, et al. The prevalence of enteric pathogens in diarrhoeic thoroughbred foals in Britain and Ireland. Equine Vet J 1991; 23:405–9.

52. Myers LL, Shoop DS, Byars TD. Diarrhea associated with enterotoxigenic Bacteroides fragilis in foals. Am J Vet Res 1987;48:1565–7.

53. Cudd T, Pauly TH. Necrotizing enterocolitis in two equine neonates. Compend Contin Educ Vet 1987;9:88–96.

54. Vaala WE. Perinatal asphyxia syndrome in foals. Comp Equine 2009;134–40.

55. Sykes BW, Hewetson M, Hepburn RJ, et al. European college of equine internal medicine consensus statement - equine gastric ulcer syndrome (EGUS) in adult horses. J Vet Intern Med 2015;29:1288–99.

56. Roberts VLH, Knottenbelt DC, Williams A, et al. Suspected primary lactose intolerance in neonatal foals. Equine Vet Educ 2008;20:249–51.

57. Weese JS, Parsons DA, Staempfli HR. Association of *Clostridium difficile* with enterocolitis and lactose intolerance in a foal. J Am Vet Med Assoc 1999;214: 229–32.

58. Nemoto M, Hata H, Higuchi T, et al. Evaluation of rapid antigen detection kits for diagnosis of equine rotavirus infection. J Vet Med Sci 2010;72:1247–50.

59. Palmer JE. Fluid therapy in the neonate: not your mother's fluid space. Vet Clin North Am Equine Pract 2004;20:63–75.

60. Magdesian KG. Fluid therapy for neonatal foals. In: Fielding CL, Magdesian KG, editors. Ames (IA): Wiley Blackwell; 2015. p. 279–300.

61. Corley KTT. Inotropes and vasopressors in adults and foals. Vet Clin Equine 2004; 20:77–106.

62. Durando MM, MacKay RJ, Linda S, et al. Effects of polymyxin B and Salmonella typhimurium antiserum on horses given endotoxin intravenously. Am J Vet Res 1994;55:921–7.

63. Tillotson K, Traub-Dargatz JL. Gastrointestinal protectants and cathartics. Vet Clin North Am Equine Pract 2003;19:599–615.

64. Weese JS, Cote NM, deGannes RVG. Evaluation of in vitro properties of di-tri-octahedral smectite on clostridial toxins and growth. Equine Vet J 2003;35: 638–41.

65. Mullen KR, Yasuda K, Divers TJ, et al. Equine faecal microbiota transplant: current knowledge, proposed guidelines and future directions. Equine Vet Edu. [Epub ahead of print].

66. Furr M, Cohen ND, Axon JE, et al. Treatment with histamine-type 2 receptor antagonists and omeprazole increase the risk of diarrhoea in neonatal foals treated in intensive care units. Equine Vet J 2012;44:s80–86.

67. Corley KTT, Hollis AR. Antimicrobial therapy in neonatal foals. Equine Vet Educ 2009;21:436–48.

68. Weese JS. Enteric clostridial infections. In: Sellon DC, Long MT, editors. Equine infectious diseases. 2nd edition. St. Louis (MO): Saunders Elsevier; 2014. p. 322–33.

69. Malorny B, Hoorfar J. Toward standardization of diagnostic PCR testing of fecal samples: lessons from the detection of salmonellae in pigs. J Clin Microbiol 2005;43:3033–7.

70. Kurowski PB, Traub-Dargatz JL, Morley PS, et al. Detection of Salmonella spp in fecal specimens by use of real-time polymerase chain reaction assay. Am J Vet Res 2002;63:1265–8.

71. Bartlett JG, Gerding DN. Clinical recognition and diagnosis of *Clostridium difficile*. Clin Infect Dis 2008;46:S12–8.

72. MedinaTorres CE, Weese JS, Staempfli HR. Validation of a commercial enzyme immunoassay for detection of *Clostridiumdifficile* toxins in feces of horses with acute diarrhea. J Vet Intern Med 2010;24:628–32.

73. Garcia LS, Shimizu RY. Evaluation of nine immunoassay kits (enzyme immunoassay and direct fluorescence) for detection of *Giardia lamblia* and *Cryptosporidium parvum* in human fecal specimens. J Clin Microbiol 1997;35:1526–9.

74. Pusterla N, Jackson R, Wilson R, et al. Temporal detection of Lawsonia intracellularis using serology and real-time PCR in Thoroughbred horses residing on a farm endemic for equineproliferative enteropathy. Vet Microbiol 2009;136:173–6.

75. Nielsen MK, Reinemeyer CR, Sellon DC. Nematodes. In: Sellon DC, Long MT, editors. Equine infectious diseases. 2nd edition. St. Louis (MO): Saunders Elsevier; 2014. p. 475–89.

76. McKenzie HC, Geor RJ. Feeding management of sick neonatal foals. Vet Clin North Am Equine Pract 2009;25:109–19.

77. Dwyer RM. Control and Prevention of Foal Diarrhea Outbreaks. In: Proceedings of the 47th Annual Convention of the American Association of Equine Practitioners. San Diego, California. November 24–28, 2001. p. 472–5.

78. Beard L. Managing foal diarrhea. Comp Equine 2009.

Diagnostics and Treatments in Chronic Diarrhea and Weight Loss in Horses

Olimpo Oliver-Espinosa, DVM, MSc, DVSc

KEYWORDS

- Horse • Chronic diarrhea • Neoplasia • Inflammatory bowel disease

KEY POINTS

- Chronic diarrhea in horses is defined as a diarrhea that has lasted several days with no improvement.
- It is the result of large intestinal diseases in the adult horse.
- Weight loss is a common finding in chronic diarrhea.
- There are many limitations to treatment of chronic diarrhea given the limited numbers in which a final diagnosis can be achieved.

Chronic diarrhea in the horse is defined as diarrhea present for more than several days with little if any improvement. There has not been consensus as to the duration of the diarrhea to become chronic. Different investigators have used different cutoff points that range from 7 days to 1 month.[1–4] Chronic diarrhea in the adult horse usually is a sign of large intestinal or colonic disease[5] and originates from a plethora of disease conditions (**Boxes 1** and **2**). These cases are usually the result of either a chronic inflammatory process or a disruption of normal physiologic homeostasis.[6] It often results in chronic weight loss.

PATIENT HISTORY

Chronic diarrhea can occur in horses of any age, sex, or breed,[7] and it has been suggested to be more common in Standardbreds.[8] The diarrhea has persisted for weeks or months.[1,3] In some cases, it is a sequela of acute diarrhea, and in other cases, there are episodes of chronic diarrhea interspersed with periods of normal feces.[1,6] Fecal consistency is reported to vary from watery to semisolid.[2–7] Weight loss is frequently reported.[2–7] Colic or recurrent colic might have occurred.[2] Deworming history may indicate an inadequate program.[2,8]

Department of Animal Health, Faculty of Veterinary Medicine and Zootechnics, National University of Colombia, Carrera 45 # 26-85, Edif. Uriel Gutiérrez, Bogotá D.C. 111321, Colombia
E-mail address: ojolivere@unal.edu.co

Vet Clin Equine 34 (2018) 69–80
https://doi.org/10.1016/j.cveq.2017.11.011
0749-0739/18/© 2017 Elsevier Inc. All rights reserved.

Box 1
Common causes of chronic diarrhea in horses

Chronic parasitism (cyathostomosis, large strongyle infection, other enteric parasites)

Salmonellosis

Equine proliferative enteropathy (*L intracellularis*)

Rodococcus equi (ulcerative enterothyphlo-colitis)

Peritonitis

Idiopathic colonic dysfunction

Inflammatory bowel disease
• Eosinophilic enteritis and multisystemic eosinophilic epitheliotropic disease
• Granulomatous enteritis
• Lymphocytic/plasmacytic enteritis/colitis
• Lymphosarcoma

Nonsteroidal anti-inflammatory drug toxicity (right dorsal colitis)

Sand enteropathy

Equine gastric ulcer syndrome

Data from Refs.[1–8]

PHYSICAL EXAMINATION

- A thorough physical examination is mandatory in the cases of chronic diarrhea because it is frequently associated with other diseases.[7]
- Rectal temperature, heart rate, and respiratory rate are frequently within normal ranges; however, some cases show pyrexia that can be persistent or intermittent.

Box 2
Less common diseases associated with chronic diarrhea

Enteroliths

Cecal impactions

Chronic intussusceptions

Pituitary pars intermedia dysfunction

Hyperlipemia

Abdominal abscess

Abdominal neoplasia

Chronic liver disease

Congestive heart failure

Pancreatic disease

Chronic renal failure

Malnutrition/starvation

Brachyspira pilosicoli

Grass sickness

Data from Refs.[2–11]

- Pyrexia occurs more commonly in inflammatory diseases, such as peritonitis, larval cyathostomiasis, chronic salmonellosis, and sand enteropathy.[2,9]
- Gastrointestinal sounds are increased in some cases due to motility abnormalities, and sand can be auscultated behind the xiphoid.[7]
- Systemic illness characterized by inappetence and depression may be present.[1,2,9]
- Weight loss is commonly observed.[1–9]
- Subcutaneous edema is common and associated with hypoalbuminemia/panhypoproteinemia, which is often caused by protein-losing enteropathy.
- Rectal examination may be without abnormal findings, but masses, colon wall thickening, or enlarged mesenteric lymph nodes may be palpated.[2,7]
- Signs of colic can be observed in some cases.[2,7,9]
- Hydration status is often normal.

DIAGNOSIS
Laboratory Examination

Clinicopathologic findings are dependent on the cause of the chronic diarrhea, but some common findings occur in most cases.

Packed cell volume and lactate can be increased in horses with dehydration, but dehydration is less frequent when compared with cases of acute diarrhea. In some cases, anemia might be present, particularly in cases of granulomatous enteritis or other inflammatory diseases.[2,9] The white blood cell count can show neutrophilia or neutropenia or can be within the reference range.[1,2,9] Fibrinogen or serum amyloid A protein (SAA) concentrations can be normal or elevated.[1,9,10] The most common abnormal clinicopathologic findings of horses with chronic diarrhea are hypoproteinemia due to hypoalbuminemia that may be accompanied by reduced, normal, or elevated globulin concentrations. On serum electrophoresis, beta-globulins may be increased in larval cyathostominosis.[1,5,6,9,10,12] Common serum electrolyte derangements are hyponatremia, hypokalemia, hypochloremia, and hypocalcemia; however, electrolyte concentrations can also be normal.[1,5,6,13,14] Acid-base abnormalities, including metabolic acidosis due to electrolyte derangements or increased lactate concentrations, can be observed. In cases with hypoalbuminemia, hypoproteinemic alkalosis is observed.[5,15] Hepatic diseases such as inflammatory diseases, fibrosis, or fatty infiltrations have been associated with chronic diarrhea. In these cases, sorbitol dehydrogenase, γ-glutamyltransferase, aspartate aminotransferase, glutamate dehydrogenase, bilirubin, and serum bile acids may be increased.[2,6] In dehydrated horses, azotemia may be seen.[6]

Abdominocentesis

Abdominocentesis should be performed in horses with hypoproteinemia or fever to rule out peritonitis, abdominal abscesses, and abdominal neoplasia.[2] In some cases of lymphosarcoma, neoplastic cells can be seen on cytologic examination[16]; however, absence of neoplastic cells does not rule out the presence of neoplasia because of the low sensitivity.[16] In cases of idiopathic eosinophilic enteritis, increased amounts of eosinophils can be seen.[17,18]

Fecal Examination

Macroscopic examination of the feces may indicate alterations in digestion or transit time within the gastrointestinal (GI) tract. Inadequate mastication, poor colonic digestion, or colonic transit time alteration should be suspected when watery feces or loose feces with long feed particles are observed.[2] Adult cyathostomes, 4th-stage larvae, or both may be observed in the feces, but microscopic examination of a wet smear of feces may be needed to see the larvae. The absence of larvae does not necessarily rule out cyathostomins as a cause of clinical disease.[19,20] Fecal egg counts are usually negative.[19] The presence of sand or gravel in the feces is not abnormal, but large amounts detected by sedimentation are highly suggestive of significant quantities in the colon.[21] White blood cells in feces have been used to assess the presence of inflammatory lesions in the intestines, but this test is more likely to be positive in horses with acute inflammatory diarrhea.[22] Fecal flotation for parasites should be performed in any horse with hypoalbuminemia weight loss and/or chronic diarrhea. Repeat examination daily for 5 days is indicated when suspecting cyathostomins to increase the likelihood of a positive result.[23] Fecal cultures should be done to rule out chronic salmonellosis. More than the 5 recommended cultures might be needed to confirm the infection.[24] Salmonella indentification by polymerase chain reaction (PCR) instead of culture should be considered to improve sensitivity; however, it should be followed up by culture to confirm chronic salmonellosis due to poor specificity of the PCR. Fecal PCR and serology are needed to diagnose *Lawsonia intracellularis*.[25]

Abdominal Ultrasonography

Transabdominal ultrasound allows detection of peritoneal effusion, abdominal masses, peritoneal abscesses, liver disease, and assessment of intestinal wall thickness.[26] Normal small intestinal wall thickness (duodenal and jejunal) is around 2 to 4 mm when the bowel is moderately distended.[27] Occasionally, lymphadenopathy can also be visualized. Transrectal ultrasound can also be used to measure the thickness of the small intestinal wall.[14] In cases of inflammatory bowel disease (IBD), small intestinal wall thickness can be increased.[10] Large colon has a normal wall thickness less than 4 mm.[28] In right dorsal colitis (RDC), the colonic wall thickness in the 12th intercostal space has been reported to be up to 13 mm.[29] For more details on abdominal ultrasound, consult the article by Nicola C. Cribb and Luis G. Arroyo's article, "Techniques and Accuracy of Abdominal Ultrasound in Gastro-Intestinal Diseases of Horses and Foals," in this issue.

Abdominal Radiology

Abdominal radiographs have been used to detect the presence of sand in the large intestine in cases of sand enteropathy. In a case series, all affected horses had sand detected by radiographs.[21] Abdominal radiography also allows detection of enteroliths in the large intestine. Sensitivity for detection is reported as 88.9% for the large colon and 61.5% for the small colon.[30]

Gastroscopy, Duodenal Endoscopy, and Biopsy

Gastroscopy is the only reliable antemortem diagnostic test to confirm equine gastric ulcer syndrome (EGUS) in the horse.[31] It can confirm or rule out gastric ulceration as a cause of the hypoproteinemia or chronic diarrhea.[5,14] A complete evaluation that includes all areas of the stomach should be performed. The technique has been previously described,[32] and further diagnostics and therapies for EGUS are discussed in this issue. In the case of suspected IBD, the duodenum should be visually evaluated by passing the endoscope through the pylorus and biopsies can be taken; 3 biopsy samples should be taken for diagnosis.[14]

Rectal Biopsy

Rectal biopsy has been described, but its merit is debated. It has been used in cases of chronic diarrhea to determine the presence of IBD and also to culture for *Salmonella* spp.[33] Samples are usually taken approximately one arm's length from the rectum. Histopathologic findings at this level of the GI system may not represent the entire GI tract. Another limitation is the lack of information on what variations can be considered normal in a rectal biopsy.[14,33,34] An experienced pathologist should evaluate the samples. Scattered neutrophils in small numbers are seen in the *lamina propria* but are not normally present within the surface epithelium or crypts in biopsies of control specimens. Therefore, when observed, they are always considered pathologic.[33] The presence of neoplastic cells confirms GI neoplasia; however, their absence does not rule out neoplasia.

Nuclear Scintigraphy

Nuclear scintigraphy with technetium-99m-labeled hexamethyl-propyleneamine oxime-labeled leukocytes has been used to evaluate small intestinal malabsorption.[35] Given the requirements of specialized equipment and the presence of some false negative results in horses with intestinal abnormality, the technique has limitations and is rarely used.[35]

Intestinal Absorption Tests

Absorption tests are used to assess the absorptive integrity of the small intestine, by measuring the efficiency of sugar absorption from the intestinal lumen.[36,37] The D-xylose absorption test or the oral glucose absorption test (OGAT) is indicated in cases of chronic diarrhea and/or weight loss with hypoproteinemia whereby an overt cause is not established.[36,37] The protocol to perform these tests is reported elsewhere.[36,37] The OGAT is a simple test to perform, but the glucose metabolism is influenced by many factors that affect test sensitivity and specificity. These factors include dietary history, gastric emptying rate, intestinal transit, age, hormonal effects, and the metabolic state of the horse.[38] The D-xylose absorption test is not dependent on hormonal or metabolic factors.[39] It can nevertheless be affected by rate of gastric emptying, intestinal motility, intraluminal bacterial overgrowth, and renal clearance.[18]

Exploratory Surgery

Exploratory surgery is a useful diagnostic tool in some cases of chronic diarrhea. During exploratory surgery, full-thickness intestinal biopsies of abnormal intestines can be taken in suspected IBD cases. Intra-abdominal abscesses and neoplasia can also be visualized.[14,18] Exploratory laparoscopy is minimally invasive, but to date it is not widely used because full-thickness biopsies are a challenge to obtain using this technique. Incisional healing may be compromised because affected horses are systemically compromised by the catabolic state and hypoproteinemia.[14]

TREATMENT
Nonspecific Therapy

If a primary cause can be established, treatment will depend mainly on this primary cause. In many cases, a primary cause cannot be established and specific treatment is not possible. General and supportive therapeutic principles should be implemented, using a problem-oriented approach to the clinical alterations.

Chronic diarrhea can result in significant enteral loss of fluid, electrolytes, and proteins. To correct these losses, intravenous fluid therapy might be necessary (see Sarah D. Shaw and Henry Stämpfli's article, "Diagnosis and treatment of undifferentiated and infectious acute diarrhea in the adult horse," in this issue, for details on fluid therapy). The horse's own voluntary intake should be monitored and subtracted from the amount administered. This measurement can be achieved by offering water from a bucket.

Hyponatremia is common in chronic diarrhea as a consequence to losses into the GI lumen. Mechanisms include sodium secretion, failure to absorb sodium in the large colon, or a combination of both.[40] Hyponatremia should be corrected using intravenous or oral fluid therapy. When severe and chronic hyponatremia is present, the rate of correction should not exceed 8 to 12 mEq/L/d to avoid the risk of osmotic demyelination syndrome.[41]

Plasma hypokalemia is also common in chronic diarrhea cases and leads to a full body depletion. Hypokalemia can be corrected by using a balanced electrolyte solution for intravenous fluid therapy and adding additional KCl as necessary. Supplemented fluids can be administrated safely if the rate of administration does not exceed 0.5 mEq/kg/h. To correct body deficits, KCl should be administered orally at 50 g twice daily for several days.[42]

Acid-base derangements are usually corrected by treating dehydration to resolve lactic acidosis and correcting electrolyte concentrations. For further information, refer to Sarah D. Shaw and Henry Stämpfli's article, "Diagnosis and treatment of undifferentiated and infectious acute diarrhea in the adult horse," in this issue.

Often horses with chronic diarrhea maintain their hydration status by increasing their water intake. In these cases, intravenous fluid therapy might not be necessary. Ad libitum water and additional oral electrolyte solution mixed with water should be offered to allow the horse to balance its own electrolyte and fluid homeostasis.

The use of probiotics has been recommended in chronic diarrhea in adult horses.[43] The use is based on purported mechanisms that include modulation of the host innate and acquired immune system, antimicrobial production, competitive exclusion, and inhibition or inactivation of bacterial toxins.[44] These mechanisms have been based on in vitro studies, but in vivo health benefits have not been proven. Probiotics are used because of their lack of severe adverse effects, ease of administration, and low cost.[44] Refer to Angelika Schoster article, "Probiotic use in equine gastrointestinal disease," in this issue, for additional details.

To reduce GI inflammation, bismuth subsalicylate (BSS) has been used. BSS is thought to decrease inflammation and secretion in the large colon and may therefore be beneficial in the treatment of equine diarrhea.[45] There are no studies in horses that support its use, and even in human medicine, there is no evidence of benefit for persistent diarrhea.[46] The use of up to 1liter/500 Kg horse q 12 hours has been recommended by extrapolating human doses,[47] but no beneficial effect has been observed in horses.[47]

Anecdotally, equine fecal microbiota transplants (FMT) using cecal contents or fresh feces from healthy horses have been used in an attempt to replace some of the normal bacterial flora of the colon.[43,45] Several important points should be considered before performing equine FMT. The donor should be clinically healthy and should not have undergone antimicrobial treatment in the recent past. Laboratory testing should be performed to reduce the risk of infectious disease transmission.[48] To obtain the transplant material, manure can be obtained by rectal evacuation or off the ground. Alternatively, cecal contents can be harvested immediately after euthanasia or from a recently expired horse. The material is mixed with warm water or isotonic saline and blended thoroughly to capture cellulolytic bacteria off long fibers. The mixture needs to be strained to allow administration via nasogastric tube.[48] The dose is 2 to 3 L via nasogastric tube for an average adult horse and 200 mL for a foal. When possible, offer free choice early-cut long-stem hay following FMT. Repeat FMT daily until improvement in fecal consistency is seen or up to 3 days.[48] There are no controlled studies evaluating FMT use in horses, and a standard protocol for FMT in horses has not been developed either. The previous recommendations are anecdotal yet. For details on the equine microbiome and FMT, see Marcio Carvalho Costa and Jeffery Scott Weese's article, "Understanding the intestinal microbiome in health and disease," in this issue.

Specific Treatments

Treatment of larval cyathostominosis is frequently unrewarding, particularly in severe cases. Mortalities of 40% to 70% despite aggressive treatment have been reported.[19,49,50] Only 2 anthelmintic drugs have shown efficacy against encysted cyathostomes: fenbendazole at either 7.5 or 10 mg/kg body weight (BW), orally, every 24 hours for 5 days and moxidectin at 400 µg/kg BW, orally.[49,51] However, there is evidence of widespread resistance to fenbedazole.[52] One important aspect when using these 2 anthelmintics in larval Cyathostominosis is the consequence of killing the inhibited stages. Fenbendazole kills inhibited stages, which results in severe inflammation, whereas no inflammation occurs when moxidectin is used.[53] Anti-inflammatories can be given at the same time as fenbendazole to try and alleviate severe signs of inflammation.

Antimicrobial therapy for the treatment of acute as well as chronic salmonellosis in horses is controversial. There is no evidence that antimicrobial therapy is beneficial in altering the course of salmonellosis in adult horses.[45] The use of antibiotics in these chronic cases should be judicious and based on antibiogram results. The aim should be prevention of systemic dissemination while supporting the natural immune response to clear the infection rather than eliminating fecal shedding or carrier states.[45] Antimicrobial administration has been shown to increase the risk of fecal shedding of *Salmonella*.[47]

The use of iodochlorhydroxyquin (clioquinol) (5–10 g orally every 24 hours) for horses with chronic nonspecific colitis or idiopathic colonic dysfunction has been suggested. This drug is used to treat skin infections and diarrhea in humans. The mechanism of action of the drug in the intestine is not known, but it is known to be a chelator of copper, iron, and zinc.[54] In horses, it is thought to modify the colonic microflora and possibly has antiprotozoal activity.[43] There are no studies to support its use.

Sulfasalazine is a colon-specific prodrug commonly used for the treatment of IBDs, such as ulcerative colitis and Crohn's disease in humans. There are also reports of its use in eosinophilic colitis in dogs and cats and typhlocolitis in horses.[55] Its exact mechanism of action is also unknown, but it is thought to have anti-inflammatory effects because of inhibition of eicosanoid metabolism, and the interaction of 5-aminosalisylic acid (5-ASA) with oxygen-derived free radicals.[54] It has been successfully used in a reported equine case at a dose regimen adapted from small animals (16 mg/kg orally once a day for 5 days, followed by 8 mg/kg orally every 24 hours for 10 days).[56]

Zinc bacitracin (10 mg/kg every 12 hours during the first 24 hours continuing once a day) has been used in chronic diarrhea with an open diagnosis. Bacitracin is not absorbed from the gut and acts mainly against gram-positive anaerobe bacteria.[57] In acute diarrhea, it has not been recommended because of a high prevalence of resistance among equine *Clostridium difficile* isolates[58]; however, it has been shown that bacitracin administration in experimental colitis results in improved fecal consistency.[59,60] In healthy animals, it can induce impaction.[59]

The treatment of IBD in horses has been unrewarding, and the long-term outcome is often disappointing in terms of full resolution.[9,13] Treatment of horses with granulomatous enteritis has commonly resulted in euthanasia.[9] Therapeutic management can be attempted through dietary modifications and medical therapy. The horse nutritional requirements should be calculated and provided through a highly digestible, well-balanced feed. Small amounts should be fed frequently to improve digestion and absorption.[14,56] Energy intake can be increased by feeding high-fat diets (5% to 10%) containing vegetable oils.[18] Constant parasite control has been advised given that even low parasite burdens are supposed to trigger intestinal inflammation in horses with IBD. Pyrantel tartrate (Strongid C) on a daily basis has been suggested to achieve this goal.[14] Given the level of current and emerging parasite resistance, this recommendation is highly questionable. A regular dewormer should be used every 6 months.[14] Metronidazole has been shown to be beneficial in treatment of Crohn's disease in humans. It may have a potential beneficial effect in horses with IBD given it is both an antibiotic and an anti-inflammatory agent.[14,18]

As an adjunctive treatment in cases with severe hypoproteinemia or suspected IBD, either prednisolone (0.5–1.0 mg/kg, orally, every 24 hours or every 12 hours) or dexamethasone (0.02–0.05 mg/kg, intravenously, intramuscularly, or orally, every 24 hours to 48 hours) can be used.[19] The dose should be tapered over the course of several weeks before attempting to discontinue administration. If clinical signs initially improve but worsen upon reduction of the corticosteroid dose or recur after the discontinuation, treatment should be reinstituted at a low dose. The treatment interval can then be gradually prolonged until the dose and interval are found that will keep the horse free of clinical signs while minimizing corticosteroid use.

Horses with multisystemic eosinophilic epitheliotropic disease have been treated with the antineoplastic drug hydroxyurea, and temporary improvement has been reported.[14] However, no beneficial effects have been observed when treated with other chemotherapeutic agents.[61] Alimentary lymphoma cases have responded favorably for 6 to 12 months when chemotherapy has been administered; however, they carry a poor prognosis for long-term survival.[14]

When the cause of chronic diarrhea is L intracellularis infection, treatment includes macrolide antimicrobials such as erythromycin phosphate (15–25 mg/kg orally every 12 hours), azithromycin (10 mg/kg orally every 24 hours), or clarithromycin (7.5 mg/kg orally every 12 hours), with or without rifampin (5 mg/kg orally every 12 hours or 10 mg/kg orally every 24 hours).[62] Alternative antimicrobials are tetracyclines, including oxytetracycline (6.6 mg/kg intravenously every 12 hours), doxycycline (10 mg/kg orally every 12 hours), or minocycline (4 mg/kg orally every 12 hours) and chloramphenicol (44–50 mg/kg orally every 8-12 hours) for 2 to 3 weeks.[63]

Sand enteropathy is treated by preventing further sand access and the use of laxatives.[21] The most effective combination used in one study was psyllium and mineral oil.[21] Mineral oil alone is not sufficient; it will pass around the sand without removing it.[64] Psyllium is often used on its own, but in one study, psyllium alone failed to increase evacuation of sand.[65] In another clinical study, the refractory cases were treated by the combination of magnesium sulfate and mineral oil.[66] Surgery is indicated without delay in horses with persistent colic.[21]

Medical treatment of chronic diarrhea associated with RDC includes discontinuation of nonsteroidal anti-inflammatory drug (NSAID) administration and dietary modifications consisting of low-bulk diet provided in several small feeds during the day.[29,67] Bulk feed should be reintroduced after a period of 3 to 6 months to allow the colon to heal. Psyllium has been used as a soluble dietary fiber, and the recommended dose is 100 g once daily for 3 to 6 months to promote the production of short-chain fatty acids, which may promote healing and repair of the colonic mucosa.[68] Controlled studies on psyllium mucilloid in horses are lacking. Metronidazole has been used to treat human patients with NSAID enteropathies. The administration of metronidazole might be of benefit to horses with RDC; however, the emerging threat of antibiotic resistance should be considered before using antimicrobial agents for noninfectious diseases.[69]

In conclusion, the diagnosis and treatment of horses with chronic diarrhea usually represent a great challenge to the clinician. There are many limitations to treatment of these patients given the limited numbers in which a final diagnosis can be achieved. The lack of knowledge of the alterations of horse microbiota during chronic diarrhea and the multiplicity of causes also make treatment challenging. A poor prognosis is often attached to chronic diarrhea, particularly in cases with neoplasia and IBD.

REFERENCES

1. Love S, Mair TS, Hillyer MH. Chronic diarrhea in adult horses: a review of 51 referred cases. Vet Rec 1992;130:217–9.
2. Mair T. Differential diagnosis and evaluation of chronic diarrhea in the adult horse. In: Mair T, Divers T, Ducharme N, editors. Manual of equine gastroenterology. London: WB Saunders; 2002. p. 427–30.
3. Merrit AM. Chronic diarrhea in horses: a summary. Vet Med 1994;363–7.
4. Merritt AM. Chronic diarrhoea. In: Robinson NE, editor. Current therapy in equine medicine. 1st edition. Philadelphia: WB Saunders; 1983. p. 216.
5. Stämpfli H, Oliver O. Chronic diarrhea and weight loss in three horses. Vet Clin Equine 2006;22:e27–35.
6. Jones SL. Chronic diarrhea. In: Smith BP, editor. Large animal internal medicine. 5th edition. St Louis(MO): ELSEVIER; 2015. p. 714–5.
7. Palmer J. Diarrhea. In: Anderson NV, editor. Veterinary gastroenterology. 2nd edition. Philadelphia: Lea & Febiger; 1992. p. 634–70.
8. Merrit AM. Chronic diarrhea: differential diagnosis and therapy. Lexington(KY): Proc 21st Annu Meet Am Assoc Eq Prat; 1975. p. 402–9.
9. Schumacher J, Edwards JF, Cohen ND. Chronic idiopathic inflammatory bowel diseases of the horse. J Vet Intern Med 2000;14:258–65.
10. Trachsel DS, Grest P, Nitzl D, et al. Diagnostische Aufarbeitung der chronischen Darmentzündung beim Pferd Schweiz. Schweiz Arch Tierheilkd 2010;152: 418–24.
11. Hampson DJ, Lester GD, Phillips ND. Isolation of Brachyspira pilosicoli from weanling horses with chronic diarrhea. Vet Rec 2006;158:661–2.
12. Love S, Escala J, Duncan J, et al. Studies on the pathogenic effects of experimental cyathostome infections in ponies. Cambridge(UK): Proceedings of Sixth International Conference, Equine Infectious Diseases; 1991. p. 149–55.
13. Barr B. Infiltrative intestinal disease. Vet Clin North Am Equine Pract 2006;22: e1–7.
14. Kalck KA. Inflammatory bowel disease in horses. Vet Clin Equine 2009;25: 303–15.
15. Gomez DE, Arroyo LG, Staempfli HR, et al. Physicochemical interpretation of acid-base abnormalities in 54 horses with acute severe colitis and diarrhea. J Vet Intern Med 2013;27:548–53.

16. Mair T, Hillyer MH. Clinical features of lymphosarcoma in the horse: 77 cases. Equine Vet Educ 1992;18:149–56.

17. Southwood LL, Kawcak CE, Trotter GW, et al. Idiopathic focal eosinophilic enteritis associated with small intestinal obstruction in 6 horses. Vet Surg 2000;29:415–9.

18. Mair T, Pearson GR, Divers TJ. Malabsorption syndromes in the horse. Equine Vet Educ 2006;18:383–92.

19. Peregrine AS, McEwen B, Bienzle D, et al. Larval cyathostominosis in horses in Ontario: an emerging disease? Can Vet J 2005;46:80–2.

20. Smets K, Shaw D, Deprez J, et al. Diagnosis of larval cyathostominosis in horses in Belgium. Vet Rec 1999;144:665–8.

21. Hart KA, Linnenkohl W, Mayer JR, et al. Medical management of sand enteropathy in 62 horses. Equine Vet J 2013;45:465–9.

22. Morris DD, Whitlock RH, Palmer JE. Fecal leukocytes and epithelial cells in horses with diarrhea. Cornell Vet 1983;73:265–74.

23. Tamzali Y. Chronic weight loss syndrome in the horse: a 60 case retrospective study. Equ Vet Edu 2006;18:286–96.

24. Palmer JE, Benson CE. Salmonella shedding in the equine. In: Snoyenbos GH, editor. Proceedings of the international symposium on salmonella. New Orleans (LA): American Association of Avian Pathologists; 1984. p. 161–4.

25. Pusterla N, Jackson R, Wilson R, et al. Temporal detection of Lawsonia intracellularis using serology and real-time PCR in Thoroughbred horses residing on a farm endemic for equine proliferative enteropathy. Vet Microbiol 2009;136:173–6.

26. Scharner D, Rotting AA, Gerlach K, et al. Ultrasonography of the abdomen in the horse with colic. Clin Tech Equine Pract 2002;1:118–24.

27. Desrochers A. Abdominal ultrasonography of normal and colicky adult horses. Paper presented at the AAEP Focus Meeting. Quebec, Canada, July 31–August 2, 2005.

28. Henry Barton M. Understanding abdominal ultrasonography in horses: which way is up? Compend Contin Educ Vet 2011;33:1–6.

29. Galvin N, Dillon H, McGovern F. Right dorsal colitis in the horse: minireview and reports on three cases in Ireland. Ir Vet J 2004;57:467–73.

30. Keller ME, Puchalski SM, Drake C, et al. Use of digital abdominal radiography for the diagnosis of enterolithiasis in equids: 238 cases (2008-2011). J Am Vet Med Assoc 2014;245:126–9.

31. Sykes BW, Hewetson M, Hepburn RJ, et al. European College of Equine Internal Medicine consensus statement - equine gastric ulcer syndrome (EGUS) in adult horses. J Vet Intern Med 2015;29:1288–99.

32. Sykes BW, Jokisalo JM. Rethinking equine gastric ulcer syndrome: part 1 – terminology, clinical signs and diagnosis. Equine Vet Educ 2014;26:543–7.

33. Lindberg R, Nygren A, Persson SGB. Rectal biopsy diagnosis in horses with clinical signs of intestinal disorders: a retrospective study of 116 cases. Equine Vet J 1996;28:275–84.

34. Plummer PJ. Malabsorptive maldigestive disorder with concurrent salmonella in a 3-year-old quarter horse. Vet Clin Equine 2006;22:85–94.

35. Menziers-Gow NJ, Weller R, Bowen IM, et al. Use of nuclear scintigraphy with 99mTc-HMPAO-labelled leucocytes to asses small intestinal malabsorption in 17 horses. Vet Rec 2003;153:457–62.

36. Roberts MC, Norman P. A re-evaluation of the D(+)xylose absorption test in the horse. Equine Vet J 1979;11:239–43.

37. Mair TS, Hillyer MH, Taylor FGR, et al. Small intestinal malabsorption in the horse: an assessment of the specificity of the oral glucose tolerance test. Equine Vet J 1991;23:344–6.
38. Jacobs K, Bolton JR. Effect of diet on the oral glucose tolerance test in the horse. J Am Vet Med Assoc 1982;180:884–6.
39. Bolton J, Merritt AM, Cimprich RE, et al. Normal and abnormal xylose absorption in the horse. Cornell Vet 1976;66:183–97.
40. Ecke P, Hodgson DR, Rose RJ. Induced diarrhea in horses. Part 1: fluid and electrolyte balance. Vet J 1998;155:149–59.
41. Sterns RH, Riggs JE, Schochet SS Jr. Osmotic demyelination syndrome following correction of hyponatremia. N Engl J Med 1986;314:1535–42.
42. Oliver OE, Stämpfli H. Acute diarrhea in the adult horse: case example and review. Vet Clin North Am Equine Pract 2006;22:73–84.
43. Mair T. General principles of treatment of chronic diarrhea in adult horses. In: Mair T, Divers T, Ducharme N, editors. Manual of equine gastroenterology. London: WB Saunders; 2002. p. 430–2.
44. Schoster A, Weese JS, Guardabassi L. Probiotic use in horses—what is the evidence for their clinical efficacy? J Vet Intern Med 2014;28:1640–52.
45. Feary DJ, Hassel DM. Enteritis and colitis in horses. Vet Clin North Am Equine Pract 2006;22:437–79.
46. Chowdhury HR, Yunus M, Zaman K, et al. The efficacy of bismuth subsalicylate in the treatment of acute diarrhoea and the prevention of persistent diarrhoea. Acta Paediatr 2001;90:605–10.
47. Naylor RJ, Dunkel B. The treatment of diarrhoea in the adult horse. Equine Vet Educ 2009;21:494–504. L.
48. Mullen KR, Yasuda K, Divers TJ, et al. Equine faecal microbiota transplant: current knowledge, proposed guidelines and future directions. Equine Vet Educ [Epub ahead of print].
49. Duncan JL, Bairden K, Abbott EM. Elimination of mucosal cyathostome larvae by five daily treatments with fenbendazole. Vet Rec 1998;142:268–71.
50. Corning S. Equine cyathostomins: a review of biology, clinical significance and therapy. Parasit Vectors 2009;2(Suppl 2):S1–6.
51. Bello T, Lanigan J. A controlled trial evaluation of three oral dosages of moxidectin against equine parasites. J Equine Vet Sci 1994;4:483–8.
52. Kaplan RM, Klei TR, Lyons ET, et al. Prevalence of anthelmintic resistant cyathostomes on horse farms. J Am Vet Med Assoc 2004;225:903–10.
53. Steinbach T, Bauer C, Sasse H, et al. Small strongyle infection: consequences of larvicidal treatment of horses with fenbendazole and moxidectin. Vet Parasitol 2006;139:115–31.
54. Bareggi SR, Cornelli U. Clioquinol: review of its mechanisms of action and clinical uses in neurodegenerative disorders. CNS Neurosci Ther 2012;18:41–6.
55. Knoll U, Strauhs P, Schusser G, et al. Study of the plasma pharmacokinetics and faecal excretion of the prodrug olsalazine and its metabolites after oral administration to horses. J Vet Pharmacol Ther 2002;25:135–43.
56. Valle E, Gandini M, Bergero D. Management of chronic diarrhea in an adult horse. J Equine Vet Sci 2013;33:130–5.
57. Collinder E, Berge GN, Grønvold B, et al. Influence of bacitracin on microbial functions in the gastrointestinal tract of horses. Equine Vet J 2000;32:345–50.
58. Baverud V, Gustafsson A, Franklin A, et al. Clostridium difficile: prevalence in horses and environment, and antimicrobial susceptibility. Equine Vet J 2003;35: 465–71.

59. Staempfli HR, Prescott JF, Carman RJ, et al. Use of bacitracin in the prevention and treatment of experimentally-induced idiopathic colitis in horses. Can J Vet Res 1992;56:233–6.
60. McCue M, Davis EG, Rush BR, et al. Dexamethasone for treatment of multisystemic eosinophilic epitheliotropic disease in a horse. J Am Vet Med Assoc 2003; 223:1320–3.
61. Platt H. Chronic inflammatory and lymphoproliferative lesions of the equine small intestine. J Comp Pathol 1986;96:671–84.
62. Pusterla N, Gebhart C. Equine proliferative enteropathy caused by Lawsonia intracellularis. Equine Vet Educ 2009;21:415–9.
63. Sampieri F, Hinchcliff KW, Toribio RE. Tetracycline therapy of Lawsonia intracellularis enteropathy in foals. Equine Vet J 2010;38:89–92.
64. Hotwagner K, Iben C. Evacuation of sand from the equine intestine with mineral oil, with and without psyllium. J Anim Physiol Anim Nutr (Berl) 2008;92:86–91.
65. Hammock P, Freeman D, Baker G. Failure of psyllium mucilloid to hasten evacuation of sand from the equine large intestine. Vet Surg 1998;27:547–54.
66. Ruohoniemi R, Kaikonen R, Raekallio M, et al. Abdominal radiography in monitoring the resolution of sand accumulations from the large colon of horses treated medically. Equine Vet J 2001;33:59–64.
67. Cohen ND. Right dorsal colitis. Equine Vet Educ 2002;14:212–9.
68. Argenzio RA. Short-chain fatty acids and glutamine: influence on mucosal transport and healing. Proc Ann Forum Am Coll Vet Intern Med 1994;12:539–41.
69. Bjarnason I, Hayllar J, MacPherson AJ, et al. Side effects of nonsteroidal anti-inflammatory drugs on the small and large intestine in humans. Gastroenterology 1993;104:1832–47.

Advances in Diagnostics and Treatments in Horses with Acute Colic and Postoperative Ileus

Megan Burke, DVM*, Anthony Blikslager, DVM, PhD

KEYWORDS

- Acute colic • Novel diagnostic biomarkers
- Systemic inflammatory response syndrome (SIRS) • Pain and motility management

KEY POINTS

- For horses with acute colic, the ability to differentiate between surgical and medical lesions early in the course of disease has a profound effect on prognosis.
- Differentiation of viable and nonviable intestine during colic surgery is of utmost importance for minimizing postoperative morbidity, and maximizing survival outcomes.
- Systemic inflammatory response syndrome plays a central role in many of the morbidities seen after colic surgery in the horse.

COLIC DIAGNOSTICS
Preoperative Diagnostics

Differentiating between medical and surgical causes of colic is one of the primary goals of the colic workup, because early surgical intervention improves the prognosis in horses requiring surgery. Despite the increasing availability of advanced diagnostics (hematologic analyses, abdominal ultrasound imaging, etc), the most accurate indicators of the need for surgery remain the presence of moderate to severe signs of abdominal pain, recurrence of pain after appropriate analgesic therapy, and absence of intestinal borborygmi.[1] Investigation of novel biomarkers, which may help to differentiate surgical lesions from those that can be managed medically, continues to be an active area of research.

Lactate

Lactate (primarily L-lactate), produced through anaerobic metabolism, is commonly increased in horses with colic. Lactate elevation during episodes of colic is primarily

---

NC State Veterinary Hospital, North Carolina State University, 1060 William Moore Drive, Raleigh, NC 27607, USA
* Corresponding author.
E-mail address: mjburke3@ncsu.edu

Vet Clin Equine 34 (2018) 81–96
https://doi.org/10.1016/j.cveq.2017.11.006
0749-0739/18/© 2017 Elsevier Inc. All rights reserved.

due to poor tissue perfusion and tissue hypoxia secondary to hypovolemia. Blood and peritoneal lactate concentrations, which should be equal in the normal horse, are commonly obtained during the colic workup. Several studies have shown a relationship between elevated blood and peritoneal lactate concentrations and the likelihood of a surgical lesion.

A recent study evaluated the use of serial measurements of blood lactate and peritoneal fluid lactate (PFL) in horses admitted to a referral hospital for colic.[2] Results showed that horses with elevated PFL at admission, and horses with PFL:blood lactate ratios of greater than 1 were significantly more likely to have strangulating lesions. Additionally, increases in PFL over time were significantly associated with a strangulating lesion. This association was especially strong in horses that had admission PFLs of greater than 4 mmol/L. The authors concluded that serial evaluation of PFL would be most useful in differentiating obstructive lesions such as ileal impactions, from true strangulating lesions during the early stages of the disease process when systemic compromise is minimal or nonexistent.[2] This retrospective study only involved a small subset of the overall colic population at 1 veterinary hospital owing to the requirement that multiple abdominal fluid samples be available. Therefore, selection bias may have confounded their results. Additionally, results may be of limited usefulness in areas where ileal impactions are uncommon.

Another recent study compared blood lactate concentrations in ponies and miniature horses (group ponies) admitted for colic with those of full-sized horses with a similar severity of disease.[3] Results showed that respiratory rate, rectal temperature, and blood lactate at admission were significantly higher in ponies than in the horse controls. The pony group had a longer mean duration of clinical signs before admission than the horse group. However, when regression analysis was used to evaluate the influence of time on lactate concentration, the differences between ponies and horses remained significant.[3] In contrast with results in the horses in this and other studies, there were no differences in lactate concentrations between ponies treated surgically versus those treated medically, or between those found to have strangulating lesions versus nonstrangulating lesions. Finally, there was also no significant difference in blood lactate concentrations between ponies that survived to discharge and those that did not.[3] Results of this work indicate that blood lactate levels should be interpreted cautiously in ponies if used as criteria for surgical intervention.

Another recent study compared 3 handheld lactate meters (Lactate-Pro [Arkray USA, MN], Lactate-Plus [Nova Biomedical, Waltham, MA], Lactate-Scout [SensLab, Leipzig GER]) with a bench top iStat analyzer (Radiometer America, Inc., Westlake, OH). Investigators evaluated whether or not lactate concentrations in blood and peritoneal fluid samples from horses with colic could be extrapolated between different analyzers.[4] All 3 handheld analyzers had good intra-analyzer reliability with the iStat machine for peritoneal fluid. However, only the Lactate-Plus showed good reliability at all blood lactate concentrations. Overall, handheld analyzers consistently reported lower lactate values in whole blood than the bench top analyzer for all lactate concentrations. Additionally, the differences between the handheld meters and the bench top analyzer varied across the range of measured values, with the differences increasing at higher lactate concentrations.[4] These results indicate that handheld lactate meters can be used reliably with equine whole blood or peritoneal fluid. However, owing to variability between devices, especially when analyzing whole blood samples, results should not be compared between different handheld meters, or between the handheld meters and bench top analyzers. Finally, practitioners using handheld devices may benefit from establishing a reference range for their specific device in a population of normal horses, before using it on clinical cases.

Acute phase proteins

There has been recent interest in the ability of acute phase proteins (APP) such as serum amyloid A (SAA), haptoglobin, and fibrinogen to enhance the clinician's ability to distinguish between different categories of colic. Fibrinogen is currently the most commonly evaluated APP in horses. However, fibrinogen is not an ideal APP for horses with acute colic owing to its wide reference range, slow response time, and minimal increases in the face of inflammatory stimuli.[5] Several recent studies have evaluated SAA as well as other APPs to see if they are more sensitive markers for differentiating horses needing surgical intervention from those that will respond to medical management. One study compared healthy control horses with those admitted to a tertiary referral hospital for colic. In that study, all control horses had SAA levels below the detection limit of the assay (SAA <5 μg/mL). Additionally, horses treated medically had significantly lower mean SAA levels (5 μg/mL) than horses in the surgically managed group (31.2 μg/mL).[5] However, although an admission SAA of greater than 5 μg/mL was significantly associated with the presence of a surgical lesion, there was substantial overlap in the range of SAA values between the medically managed group (<5.00–429.65 μg/mL) and those requiring surgical intervention (5–2113 μg/mL). This indicates that SAA alone could not determine the need for surgery in this study.

Another study showed that horses with inflammatory causes of colic or strangulating obstructions had significantly higher SAA levels at hospital admission than horses with simple obstructions. However, the interpretation of SAA levels in this study was complicated by the fact that values were highly dependent on the duration of colic. Additionally, substantial overlap in the range of SAA values was found between groups, reinforcing previous work showing that SAA alone cannot be used to distinguish lesion type.[6] In another study from the same group, a multivariable model including clinical parameters at admission was used to differentiate between inflammatory causes of medical colic, such as colitis, and surgical cases of colic. Of the APPs evaluated (SAA, haptoglobin, and fibrinogen) only SAA improved the sensitivity of the model for detection of horses requiring surgery. The results of this study showed also that horses with inflammatory causes of medical colic had a higher SAA levels than horses with surgical colic.[7] This finding is consistent with results of an earlier study,[8] suggesting some consistency in this finding. The clinical relevance of increased model sensitivity means that inclusion of SAA during the colic workup may result in a decreased likelihood that horses with medical colic would be incorrectly classified as needing surgery. Nonetheless, SAA values should be interpreted carefully in the context of a full medical examination based on the high degree of overlap between categories of colic patients.

A recent study evaluated the efficacy of SAA for predicting the development of postoperative complications in horses treated surgically for colic.[9] For horses in this study, SAA reached peak concentrations 24 hours before peak fibrinogen concentrations were seen. Additionally, a significant relationship between SAA concentration and the development of complications was noted between 48 and 72 hours postoperatively. However, the average time between surgery and clinical recognition of postoperative complications was 48 hours. Therefore, by the time SAA values became predictive, postoperative complications were often already apparent clinically, making SAA of limited added value in predicting complications after colic surgery.

Another study evaluated SAA as a noninvasive way to diagnose equine grass sickness (EGS).[10] SAA concentrations were compared between 4 groups: horses with EGS (based on intestinal biopsy or necropsy results), horses grazing the same pasture as EGS horses (cograzers), horses with colic, and healthy control horses. The EGS group was further divided into subgroups based on the duration of clinical signs: acute EGS (<48 hours duration), subacute EGS (2–7 days duration), and chronic EGS (>7 days duration). In this study, SAA concentrations in horses with EGS (regardless of subgroup) and inflammatory causes of colic (enteritis, colitis, peritonitis) were significantly higher than concentrations in healthy horses, cograzers, or horses with noninflammatory types of colic. These results indicate that SAA can be used to differentiate EGS from surgical colic. However, SAA cannot be used to differentiate horses with EGS from those with an inflammatory cause of colic.

Thromboelastography

Thromboelastography (TEG) is a point-of-care assay that provides information about clot formation, maturation, and lysis. One recent study evaluated the relationship between TEG parameters at admission and lesion type.[11] Relationships between TEG parameters and the development of systemic inflammatory response syndrome (SIRS), postoperative complications, and mortality were also evaluated. Once activation and consumption of clotting factors has begun, traditional coagulation tests cannot differentiate between hypercoagulable and hypocoagulable states. The aim of this study was to determine whether TEG could provide more detailed information on the balance between factor activation and consumption. Overall, 80 horses were identified as having coagulopathies. In the majority of cases, changes in TEG parameters were consistent with hypocoagulation and hypofibrinolysis. Significant associations were found between changes in TEG parameters and development of SIRS, diarrhea, thrombophlebitis, laminitis, and nonsurvival. However, no single TEG parameter was found to predict outcome for horses with colic.[11] Therefore, although TEG was found to be an improvement over traditional coagulation testing, great interhorse variability in TEG parameters was noted, which makes interpretation and clinical use difficult. In addition, the use of nonsteroidal antiinflammatory drugs (NSAIDs) (a common therapeutic intervention in horses with colic) may affect the results of TEG, owing to their inhibitory effects on platelet function via the cyclooxygenase (COX)-1 pathway. This potential interaction should be investigated before clinical application of TEG.

Alcohol dehydrogenase

Alcohol dehydrogenase (ADH) has recently shown promise as a marker of intestinal ischemia in an experimental rat model.[12] In a recent equine study, serum ADH activity was evaluated in horses with acute abdominal obstruction to determine the diagnostic and prognostic usefulness of the enzyme for differentiating horses with strangulating lesions.[13] ADH activity was compared between a control group of healthy horses and horses admitted to a university teaching hospital with signs of colic. Blood samples in colic horses were drawn before beginning any therapeutic intervention. The study found that ADH activity was significantly greater in horses with any type of colic than in control horses. Additionally, ADH activity levels were significantly different between horses with a nonstrangulating obstruction, and those with any type of strangulating lesion. An optimal cutoff for identifying strangulating lesions was set at an ADH concentration of 20 U/L, which yielded a sensitivity and specificity of 80.5% and 80.6%, respectively. Conversely, nonsurvival was associated with an ADH activity of greater than 80 U/L.

In this study, ADH activity was quantified using a spectrophotometer, which provides relatively quick results. Therefore, this methodology may provide important information in a clinically relevant time frame. Although the results of this work are promising, ADH activity should be compared with other variables currently used to predict survival and lesion type in horses with colic before it is used for clinical decision making.

Intraoperative Diagnostics

Pelvic flexure biopsy

In horses with large colon volvulus (LCV), there has been a great deal of interest in improving the ability to determine the level of colonic injury at surgery in an attempt to improve the ability to more accurately determine prognosis. This is because the large colon is typically twisted at least 360° at the base of the colon, beyond the limits of surgical resection. Some authors have argued that large colon resection remains beneficial nonetheless, because they are essentially "debulking" the injured colon, which will likely contribute to the sepsis and systemic inflammation postoperatively.[14] However, it is unknown whether resection of the large colon improves survival in horses with LCV. For example, in a recent study on factors associated with survival in horses with LCV, Gonzalez and colleagues[15] could show no benefit of resection. One possibility is that it is the preoperative absolute level of injury sustained throughout the colonic mucosa, and not resection, that ultimately determines a horse's likelihood of survival. In studies assessing frozen sections of the large colon on an emergency basis, large colon biopsy was found to be significantly associated with survival.[16] However, given that veterinary hospitals do not typically have the ability to read histologic sections on an emergency basis, the practicality of pelvic flexure biopsies is limited. Nonetheless, assessment of biopsies may still be instructive for updating the prognosis in the postoperative period, given that the critical care of a horse recovering from surgery for an LCV can be protracted and very expensive. In addition, there is hope that some colonic tissue parameters such as the degree of mucosal hemorrhage may be assessed patient side in the future. For instance, in the study by Gonzalez and colleagues,[15] the most useful parameter on a colonic biopsy for determining prognosis was hemorrhage score (**Fig. 1**). Given that this score is essentially an estimate of the level of color change (red) present within tissues with increasing levels of injury, it may be possible to develop an assay capable of measuring color on homogenized colonic mucosa. A hemorrhage score of greater than 3 out of 4

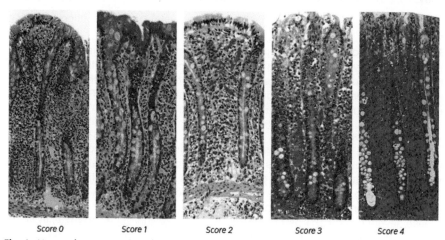

Score 0   Score 1   Score 2   Score 3   Score 4

Fig. 1. Hemorrhage score in colon volvulus. Histologic sections denoting grades 1 to 4 hemorrhage score in the mucosa of horses with naturally occurring large colon volvulus. Horses with a hemorrhage score of 4 were significantly more likely to be euthanized or die as compared with horses with a score of 3 or less [H&E, original magnification ×40]. (*Adapted from* Gonzalez LM, Fogle CA, Baker WT, et al. Operative factors associated with short-term outcome in horses with large colon volvulus: 47 cases from 2006 to 2013. Equine Vet J 2015;47:280; with permission.)

(see **Fig. 1**) resulted in an 8.8-fold increased risk of mortality, supporting the potential clinical significance of assessment of mucosal hemorrhage. Furthermore, with digital analysis of a hemorrhage area, the assessment of survival was even more accurate.[15] Nonetheless, more work is required to make this practical for use by colic surgeons. Furthermore, caution should be exercised when evaluating a single study. For example, in another recent study, histologic scoring of pelvic flexure biopsies did not accurately predict survival in horses with LCV, whereas heart rate and packed cell volvulus 24 hours after surgery were significantly associated with survival.[17]

Dark field microscopy
A recent study evaluated dark field microscopy to assess colon viability in horses with naturally occurring surgical lesions of the large colon. Microperfusion, which has previously been correlated to tissue viability,[18] was measured after lesion correction using a handheld, digital dark field microscope fitted with a sterile tip.[19] Dark field microscopy images were compared with concurrently obtained pelvic flexure biopsy samples. A significant relationship was found between increasing severity of histologic score, and decreasing perfused vessel density (PVD). Additionally, a significant decrease in PVD was seen in horses with strangulating lesions (eg, LCV), compared with horses with simple obstructions (eg, enterolith, feed impaction), and control horses. Although PVD in strangulating lesions was consistently lower than in nonstrangulating obstructions (eg, colon displacements), the difference was not significant. Image acquisition took a mean of 4.3 minutes, with image processing to obtain PVD scores taking 40 minutes, and requiring an experienced operator.[18] A minimum total turnaround time of 45 to 60 minutes is a substantial improvement over the 5-day turnaround time for pelvic flexure biopsy. However, it is still at the upper limit of what is reasonable in a clinical setting. The results of this study have shown that there are differences in PVD between different kinds of surgical lesions of the large colon. If further research can define a "cutoff" value for PVD that can differentiate a viable and nonviable colon, this technique may prove to have concrete future clinical applications.

Postoperative Diagnostics
SIRS is implicated in many of the postoperative complications that lead to morbidity after colic surgery. Diagnosis of SIRS is generally based on recognition of 1 or more clinical signs associated with the syndrome. Early recognition and therapeutic intervention lead to decreased morbidity and higher rates of survival. Therefore, recent research has focused on additional ways to recognize SIRS.

Lactate and cardiac troponin 1
Cardiac troponin 1 (cTn1) assays are used to diagnose myocardial infarction in humans. Additionally, this assay is also used as a prognostic indicator in critically ill patients with a variety of disease processes. Most equine studies have focused on cTn1 in relation to exercise, or in horses with suspected toxicoses. A recent prospective study compared concentrations of lactate, which are commonly used to indicate disease severity, and cTn1 as prognostic indicators of survival in horses with acute gastrointestinal disease.[20] No significant difference in preoperative concentrations of either lactate or cTn1 was found between survivors and nonsurvivors. There was a significant increase in postoperative lactate concentrations in nonsurvivors at 24 and 72 hours postoperatively, but not at 12 or 48 hours. Conversely, cTn1 levels were found to be significantly increased at all time points postoperatively (12, 24, 48, and 72 hours) in nonsurvivors, when compared with surviving horses.[20] Increased cTn1 concentrations in nonsurvivors are likely due to myocardial damage secondary

to severe sepsis and inflammation. Results of this study have indicated that serial cTn1 assays may have clinical value as predictors of survival in the early postoperative period, and may complement information gained by serial lactate measurements.

Blood granulocytes, plasma myeloperoxidase, and plasma elastase

Tissue injury that occurs as part of the pathogenesis of acute abdominal disease, as well as injury secondary to surgical intervention, results in neutrophil activation. Cytokines such as myeloperoxidase (MPO) and elastase released during neutrophil activation can lead to SIRS, resulting in increased postoperative morbidity and decreased survival. A recent study examined time trends of blood granulocyte counts, plasma MPO, and elastase concentrations during the perioperative period in relation to type of surgical procedure, development of postoperative ileus, and overall outcome. Results showed that horses that developed ileus had significantly lower granulocyte counts than those that did not develop ileus. In addition, granulocyte counts were significantly lower for 4.25 days postoperatively, and MPO concentrations were significantly higher for 6.25 days postoperatively in nonsurvivors compared with survivors.[21] However, owing to high levels of variability, MPO concentrations had to be log transformed before statistical analysis. Therefore, unlike granulocyte counts, MPO values cannot be used alone as a prognostic indicator of survival in horses.

COLIC TREATMENT
Preoperative Treatment

Hypertonic saline versus pentastarch

Studies have shown a significant association between packed cell volume (PCV) on admission, and postoperative survival in horses with surgical lesions admitted to referral hospitals for colic. A recent prospective, randomized study evaluated reduction in PCV, and long-term survival in horses administered either hypertonic saline (HS), or pentastarch before undergoing exploratory laparotomy for colic. Only horses with a PCV of 46 or greater were included. Horses were not given sedation or additional fluid therapy during HS or pentastarch administration. Both treatments produced a significant decrease in PCV compared with preadministration values. However, HS decreased PCV twice as much as did pentastarch, which was statistically significant.[22] Although survival was equivalent across treatments, the relative affordability of HS, and the potential for complications associated with synthetic colloid administration make HS a logical choice when rapid volume resuscitation is needed in horses with acute colic requiring surgical intervention.

Antibiotic dose and timing

Prophylactic antimicrobial administration has been shown to decrease the incidence of surgical site infection in both human and veterinary medicine. Guidelines in the human literature outlining the selection and administration of prophylactic antimicrobials have been in place for the last 20 years,[23] and are generally extrapolated to veterinary patients. A recent equine study evaluated adherence to accepted prophylactic guidelines in horses undergoing colic surgery, and proposed an equine-specific set of guidelines for horses undergoing surgery for colic (**Box 1**). Overall, only 11.6% of horses in this study population received the appropriate dose of antimicrobials within 60 minutes of the surgical incision. The most common dosing error was underdosing, and the most common timing error was administering antimicrobials more than 60 minutes before making the incision. Additionally, 63.7% of horses should have been redosed with a time-dependent antimicrobial (most commonly potassium penicillin) intraoperatively. Owing to these results, protocols have been put in place at this

---

Box 1
Suggested guidelines for antimicrobial prophylaxis in patients undergoing clean-contaminated surgical procedures

- Antimicrobials are indicated for all clean-contaminated surgical procedures.
- Antimicrobial selection should be based on efficacy against common bacterial contaminants for the type of procedure performed.
- Broad-spectrum antimicrobials are recommended, but prophylactic therapy should consist of lower generation drugs, in an effort to minimize the emergence of resistant bacterial strains.
- Antimicrobials should be administered intravenously, ideally within 30 to 60 minutes before the first surgical incision.
- Patients should be redosed intraoperatively if surgery is still ongoing 2 half-lives after the preoperative dose.
- Standard aseptic technique and infection control measures should be rigorously followed during clean-contaminated procedures; antimicrobial therapy should not be expected to compensate for poor technique.

---

hospital to improve adherence to accepted guidelines now enabling collection of prospective data to investigate the results of these protocols.[24] The problems associated with appropriate prophylactic antimicrobial administration identified in this study highlight the importance of establishing protocols in veterinary medicine to ensure that antimicrobials are administered in accordance with an evidence-based approach to ensure optimal outcomes for patients.

INTRAOPERATIVE TREATMENT
Effect of Temperature on Motility

Studies in mice have shown that smooth muscle contractility is highly temperature dependent.[25] Exteriorization of bowel during surgery, as well as lavage with room temperature fluids may cause a decrease in temperature of equine small intestine during exploratory laparotomy. A recent in vitro study investigated the effect of changes in temperature on smooth muscle contractility in the equine ileum.[26] Frequency, duration, amplitude and resting membrane potential were measured as temperature was decreased from 37°C to 27°C. Segments were then returned to a temperature of 37°C before the temperature being increased to 41°C. A significant linear relationship was found between bowel temperature and frequency of slow waves, with frequency increasing or decreasing by 0.5 cycles per minute for every 1°C increase or decrease. Slow wave amplitude and resting membrane potential of the cells were not affected by changes in temperature.[26] Interestingly, it was noted that the frequency of slow waves returned to baseline once cooled bowel was returned to 37°C. This work indicates that temperature does affect bowel motility in equine small intestine. This was an in vitro study; therefore, the relevance of these results on the development of ileus or other postoperative complications is unknown. However, it seems prudent to use warm lavage fluid, and to minimize the amount of time that bowel is exteriorized intraoperatively.

Effect of Lidocaine on Motility

Lidocaine is most commonly used postoperatively to prevent or treat postoperative ileus. Several recent studies have investigated the effect of lidocaine on jejunal contractility at the time of, as well as after ischemia and reperfusion (IR) injury. In 1 study, lidocaine was shown to significantly improve motility in jejunal segments after IR injury.[27] However, contractility was significantly better in IR-injured segments from horses that had also received lidocaine intravenously at the time of IR injury, compared with those that had not. Additional work by the same group compared the effects of lidocaine on contractility of control and IR-injured segments of jejunum.[28] Lidocaine produced a significant increase in the frequency of contractions in both control and IR-injured segments. However, a higher concentration of lidocaine was needed in IR-injured segments to elicit a significant increase in frequency of contractions. Taken together, these studies suggest that the intraoperative administration of lidocaine at the time of reperfusion injury may improve the response of small intestine to postoperative administration. However, they also imply that IR injury may have a detrimental effect on smooth muscle response to lidocaine. It should be noted that these studies were a combination of in vivo and in vitro models. Additionally, the amount of lidocaine used to incubate jejunal segments was greater than that used clinically.

POSTOPERATIVE COMPLICATIONS
Endotoxemia

Detecting endotoxin
The detection of endotoxemia has been troublesome because of the difficulty of running assays such as the limulus amebocyte lysate assay on a clinical basis, and also because it is assumed that there are intermittent "showers" of lipopolysaccharide (LPS) across injured mucosa that may make detection of LPS inconsistent. Therefore, investigators have searched for alternate means of detecting endotoxemia, or have relied on clinical parameters such as heart rate to classify horses as "endotoxemic."[29]

A recent study assessed soluble CD14 (sCD14), a molecule that is consistently related to the onset of endotoxemia, and is released into circulation (**Fig. 2**).[30] sCD14 is released by macrophages to bind LPS in response to Toll-like receptor 4 signaling via nuclear factor kappa B. This is in contrast with membrane-bound CD14, which complexes with Toll-like receptor 4 to bind LPS at the surface of the cell. It is thought that sCD14 serves to amplify the cellular "alarm" signals. Interestingly, in a study on sCD14 in horses with colic classified as either endotoxemic or non-endotoxemic (using clinical parameters of heart rate >70 beats/min, PCV >45%, and/or a lesion likely to result in endotoxemia), there was a close correlation between sCD14 concentrations and clinical evidence of endotoxemia.[30] Conversely, no correlation could be found between LPS concentrations as measured by the limulus amebocyte lysate assay and the clinical evidence of endotoxemia.

Treating endotoxemia
Clinical signs associated with endotoxemia in horses are the result of inflammatory mediators synthesized by the horse's cells, rather than damage caused by the LPS molecule itself.[31] Because horses mount an excessive inflammatory response in the face of LPS, NSAIDs are the most commonly administered medications used to combat the clinical signs of endotoxemia. However, owing to their relative lack of specificity, NSAIDs can cause harmful side effects, even within the published therapeutic ranges. Therefore, discovery of new and hopefully more specific compounds to combat endotoxemia is an active area of research.

A recent study investigated the ability of lidocaine to reduce signs of experimental endotoxemia.[32] Horses received 500 ng/kg of LPS via intraperitoneal injection, followed by a constant rate infusion of either saline (control) or lidocaine. Lidocaine was found to significantly decrease the clinical signs associated with endotoxemia.

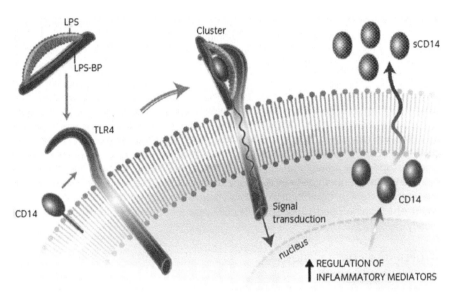

Fig. 2. Generation of soluble CD14 (sCD14) in horses in response to lipopolysaccharide (LPS). sCD14 is released by macrophages in response to binding of LPS, and may be indicative of the relative level of endotoxemia in horses. LPS-BO, lipopolysaccharide binding protein; TLR4, Toll-like receptor 4. (*From* Fogle J, Jacob M, Blikslager A, et al. Comparison of lipopolysaccharides and soluble CD14 measurement between clinically endotoxaemic and nonendotoxaemic horses. Equine Vet J 2017;49(2):156; with permission.)

There were no differences in hematologic parameters or mean arterial pressure between groups, but horses in the lidocaine group had significantly lower serum and peritoneal concentrations of tumor necrosis factor (TNF)-α, a major proinflammatory cytokine associated with endotoxemia, as compared with control horses. Although lidocaine is most commonly used as a prokinetic after colic surgery, results of this study indicate that it may have an antiinflammatory role in horses with clinical signs of endotoxemia.

Another recent study compared the efficacy of ethyl pyruvate (EP) and flunixin meglumine (FM) for decreasing clinical signs and proinflammatory gene expression in horses receiving intravenous endotoxin. Horses that received either EP or FM had significantly lower pain scores than horses that did not receive treatment with either drug (controls). Horses receiving EP had significantly higher rectal temperatures 90 minutes after administration of LPS than either control horses or horses receiving FM. Both EP and FM treatments significantly reduced TNF-α concentrations compared with controls.[33] EP was inferior to FM at suppressing fever, but showed equivalent efficacy at decreasing signs of pain associated with LPS. Additionally, EP showed a superior ability to decrease production of interleukin-6, a proinflammatory cytokine that may contribute to postoperative ileus.

A second recent study also investigated the antiinflammatory properties of EP, rolipram (a phosphodiesterase inhibitor), azithromycin, and metformin in equine whole blood samples exposed to LPS. All 4 drugs caused a concentration-dependent decrease in TNF-α production, with rolipram, azithromycin, and EP also causing a concentration-dependent inhibition of interleukin-1β production.[34] Although EP was not the most potent inhibitor of either TNF-α or interleukin-1β, it did show substantial inhibition of both cytokines at concentrations previously shown to be both efficacious and safe.[33] Although additional work would be needed to identify the appropriate dosing interval of EP in horses, the results of these 2 studies indicate that EP may have promise for treatment of the clinical signs of endotoxemia in horses.

Polymyxin B is commonly used to treat endotoxemia, because it binds the lipid A moiety of the LPS molecule in a 1:1 ratio. At doses of greater than 6000 U/kg, polymyxin B can cause toxic owing to its ability to disrupt phospholipid membranes. A recent study evaluated the effects of multiple doses of polymyxin B on serum concentrations of the drug, as well as on renal function.[35] For this study, horses were administered a single dose of 6000 U/kg in 1 L of saline over 15 minutes. After a 2-week washout period, the same horses received 6000 U/kg in 1 L of saline over 15 minutes at 8-hour intervals for a total of 5 doses. Concentrations of polymyxin B in serum were evaluated for 24 hours after the last dose of polymyxin. In addition, the urine gamma-glutamyl transferase-to-creatinine ratio was calculated for each horse, as a measure of kidney function. Finally, blood from each horse was incubated with LPS in vitro to evaluate the anti-LPS activity of polymyxin B after single dose and repeat infusion.

Pharmacokinetic analysis showed that serum concentrations of greater than 0.20 μg/mL were needed to neutralize 75% of LPS activity. A dose of 6000 U/kg given every 8 hours was found to keep serum concentrations of polymyxin B above this threshold. No alterations in the gamma-glutamyl transferase-to-creatinine ratio were seen in any horse, indicating that this dose and dosing interval do not result in toxicosis. Finally, there was no evidence of buildup of polymyxin B in serum after repeated dosing. The results of this study provide good information about the safety and efficacy of polymyxin B in the treatment of endotoxemia. However, several points should be considered. First, this study was performed in healthy horses; therefore, results may not be applicable in clinically endotoxemic horses. Second, because the toxicity of polymyxin B results from interactions with cell membranes, studies evaluating the accumulation of the drug in organ tissue after repeated administrations are critical to truly understanding the potential for toxicity with repeat administration.

Di-tri-octahedral smectite (Bio Sponge), a natural clay, is commonly used to improve fecal consistency in horses with colitis. Additionally, it may have potential as an antiendotoxic treatment by acting as a mechanical barrier, reducing translocation of gram-negative bacteria from the lumen of the gut. Recently, the efficacy of Bio Sponge to reduce both the incidence of diarrhea, and the clinical signs of endotoxemia in horses treated surgically for disease of the large intestine was evaluated prospectively.[36] Horses admitted to a veterinary teaching hospital with surgical disease of the large colon were enrolled, and randomly assigned to receive either Bio Sponge or placebo treatment postoperatively.

Significantly fewer horses in the Bio Sponge grouped developed postoperative diarrhea compared with the placebo group. However, no difference in the clinical parameters associated with endotoxemia was noted between groups. This study provides support for the use of Bio Sponge postoperatively in horses with surgical lesions of the large intestine. However, further study into any antiendotoxic effects of Bio Sponge are warranted.

Pain Management

With the advent of COX-2 preferential or selective inhibitors for use in horses (eg, meloxicam and firocoxib, respectively), there has been interest in the place of these medications in equine practice. In general, when treating conditions related to the gastrointestinal tract, it intuitively makes sense to use NSAIDs that are more selective to allow for the continued production of prostanoids such as prostaglandin E_2, which are known to be protective of the mucosa.[37,38] One particular advantage of COX-2 preferential or selective drugs has been their ability to allow more rapid repair of ischemic-injured mucosal as compared with the nonselective NSAID FM.[39,40] However, one concern has been the ability of these medications to treat abdominal pain as well as nonselective nonsteroidal antiinflammatory drugs, such as FM.[41] In preclinical trials comparing flunixin and meloxicam or flunixin and firocoxib, all of the medications had the same level of efficacy at reducing behavioral pain scores in horses.[39,40] An ongoing randomized clinical trial comparing FM (1.1 mg/kg, every 12 hours intravenously) with firocoxib (0.27 mg/kg loading dose; 0.09 mg/kg, every 24 hours intravenously) in horses admitted to 3 veterinary teaching hospitals for small intestinal strangulating obstruction has shown the same level of pain control for both medications (Blikslager AT, Cook VL, Southwood L, Grayson Jockey Club Research Foundation, 2017). Whether or not there are additional advantages of the COX-2 inhibitor firocoxib will require completion of the study. However, it should be noted that an off-label loading dose of firocoxib is now recommended based on research showing the need to increase the dosage to attain therapeutic levels with the first dose.[42] Alternatively, in a randomized clinical trial comparing FM (1.1 mg/kg every 12 hours intravenously) and meloxicam (0.6 mg/kg every 12 hours intravenously) in horses admitted to 3 veterinary referral hospitals, there was a significant difference in the ability of the 2 medications to control pain in that horses receiving meloxicam were significantly more likely to show gross signs of pain.[43] The study did not show any other differences between treatment groups, although there was a trend toward higher survival in the meloxicam group, which would have taken a larger study population to explore definitively.[43]

Lidocaine for Postoperative Ileus

Recent surveys both in Europe and the United States have shown that lidocaine is the preferred "promotility" agent used for horses diagnosed with postoperative ileus,[44] although the mechanisms of action in this context continue to be elusive. There is much debate regarding whether lidocaine has direct promotility effects, or if it indirectly affects motility owing to its antiinflammatory properties. Several studies have shown that lidocaine has an antiinflammatory mechanism. In preclinical studies conducted on horses with experimental strangulating obstruction of the small intestine, mucosal lesions repaired more rapidly in horses that received constant rate infusion of lidocaine after an initial loading dose,[45] and this finding was linked to significant reductions in infiltrating neutrophils.[46] However, this effect was only seen in the presence of flunixin (1.1 mg/kg every 12 hours), which seems to be the cause of reduced mucosal repair and infiltration of neutrophils.[46] In other words, detectable mucosal side effects of FM were ameliorated with concurrent administration of lidocaine. Interestingly, lidocaine does not have direct effects on either the adhesion or reactive oxygen metabolite-generating capacity of equine neutrophils,[47] suggesting some other effect on tissues that has not yet been identified. In addition, although there is the possibility that any positive effects of lidocaine on postoperative ileus might be related to a reduction in inflammation, this supposition has not been proven. Nonetheless, it is known that neutrophils migrate through intestinal tissues with surgical trauma, and do gather adjacent to ganglia within the myenteric plexus.[48]

Several recent clinical trials have attempted to evaluate the effectiveness of lidocaine for prevention of postoperative ileus. One study analyzed the association between a variety of preoperative, intraoperative, and postoperative variables on the development of postoperative ileus, as well as the influence of postoperative lidocaine treatment on the incidence or postoperative ileus and survival to discharge.[49] Interestingly, the overall frequency of developing postoperative ileus was not significantly different between horses with strangulating and nonstrangulating lesions. However, there was a significant difference in the development of postoperative ileus between the lidocaine group (21%) and the nonlidocaine group (51%). Additionally, horses that received lidocaine were 3.3 times more likely to survive to discharge than horses not treated with lidocaine, and this difference was statistically significant.[49] It should be noted that some horses received metoclopramide as well as lidocaine. However, during regression analysis, metoclopramide administration was not found to be associated with a lesser likelihood of developing postoperative ileus. This may be due to the fact that, in this study, metoclopramide was given intramuscularly at a lower dose than typically used in an effort to avoid the development of extrapyramidal signs. Additionally, this was a retrospective study and, therefore, suffers from the limitations inherent in all such studies. However, the results of this study indicate that regardless of the mechanism of action, lidocaine seems to reduce the risk of postoperative ileus, as well as improve survival to discharge.

A second study evaluated whether the routine use of lidocaine has had any effect on the prevalence, duration or total volume of postoperative reflux (POR) in horses after laparotomy for colic. This study evaluated 2 cohorts. Horses in the first cohort (2004–2006) were admitted at a time when postoperative lidocaine was infrequently used, and horses in the second cohort (2012–2014) were admitted after lidocaine use had become routine. The prevalence of POR was significantly higher in the second cohort compared with the first. There was no significant difference in prevalence, duration, or total volume of reflux between horses that received lidocaine and those that did not. Additionally, there was no significant difference in long-term survival between horses that received postoperative lidocaine and those that did not.[50] This study has several limitations. First, there has been a move in the last several years toward leaving compromised but viable bowel in situ rather than performing resection and anastomosis. The effect of leaving inflamed bowel in the abdomen on the development of POR has not been investigated, and may have confounded evaluation of the effectiveness of lidocaine. Additionally, the decision to use lidocaine was not random. Horses thought to be at increased risk of POR were more likely to be given lidocaine, again confounding the true effect of lidocaine on the prevention of POR.

Although the results of these 2 studies are contradictory, they both highlight the need for prospective, blinded, randomized, clinical trials that can truly evaluate the effectiveness of lidocaine for prevention of postoperative ileus. Until those studies are performed, the effectiveness of lidocaine as a prokinetic (whether by direct or indirect mechanisms) will remain controversial.

REFERENCES

1. White NA, Elward A, Moga KS, et al. Use of web-based data collection to evaluate analgesic administration and the decision for surgery in horses with colic. Equine Vet J 2005;37:347–50.

2. Peloso JG, Cohen ND. Use of serial measurements of peritoneal fluid lactate concentration to identify strangulating intestinal lesions in referred horses with signs of colic. J Am Vet Med Assoc 2012;240:1208–17.

3. Dunkel B, Kapff JE, Naylor RJ, et al. Blood lactate concentrations in ponies and miniature horses with gastrointestinal disease. Equine Vet J 2013;45:666–70.

4. Nieto JE, Dechant JE, le Jeune SS, et al. Evaluation of 3 handheld portable analyzers for measurement of L-lactate concentrations in blood and peritoneal fluid of horses with colic. Vet Surg 2015;44:366–72.

5. Westerman TL, Foster CM, Tornquist SJ, et al. Evaluation of serum amyloid A and haptoglobin concentrations as prognostic indicators for horses with colic. J Am Vet Med Assoc 2016;248:935–40.

6. Pihl TH, Scheepers E, Sanz M, et al. Influence of disease process and duration on acute phase proteins in serum and peritoneal fluid of horses with colic. J Vet Intern Med 2015;29:651–8.

7. Pihl TH, Scheepers E, Sanz M, et al. Acute-phase proteins as diagnostic markers in horses with colic. J Vet Emerg Crit Care (San Antonio) 2016;26:664–74.

8. Vandenplas ML, Moore JN, Barton MH, et al. Concentrations of serum amyloid A and lipopolysaccharide-binding protein in horses with colic. Am J Vet Res 2005; 66:1509–16.

9. Daniel AJ, Leise BS, Burgess BA, et al. Concentrations of serum amyloid A and plasma fibrinogen in horses undergoing emergency abdominal surgery. J Vet Emerg Crit Care (San Antonio) 2016;26:344–51.

10. Copas VE, Durham AE, Stratford CH, et al. In equine grass sickness, serum amyloid A and fibrinogen are elevated, and can aid differential diagnosis from non-inflammatory causes of colic. Vet Rec 2013;172:395.

11. Epstein KL, Brainard BM, Gomez-Ibanez SE, et al. Thrombelastography in horses with acute gastrointestinal disease. J Vet Intern Med 2011;25:307–14.

12. Gumaste UR, Joshi MM, Mourya DT, et al. Alcohol dehydrogenase: a potential new marker for diagnosis of intestinal ischemia using rat as a model. World J Gastroenterol 2005;11:912–6.

13. Gomaa N, Uhlig A, Schusser GF. Effect of Buscopan compositum on the motility of the duodenum, cecum and left ventral colon in healthy conscious horses. Berl Munch Tierarztl Wochenschr 2011;124:168–74.

14. Ellis CM, Lynch TM, Slone DE, et al. Survival and complications after large colon resection and end-to-end anastomosis for strangulating large colon volvulus in seventy-three horses. Vet Surg 2008;37:786–90.

15. Gonzalez LM, Fogle CA, Baker WT, et al. Operative factors associated with short-term outcome in horses with large colon volvulus: 47 cases from 2006 to 2013. Equine Vet J 2015;47:279–84.

16. Van Hoogmoed L, Snyder JR, Pascoe JR, et al. Use of pelvic flexure biopsies to predict survival after large colon torsion in horses. Vet Surg 2000;29:572–7.

17. Levi O, Affolter VK, Benak J, et al. Use of pelvic flexure biopsy scores to predict short-term survival after large colon volvulus. Vet Surg 2012;41:582–8.

18. Kerger H, Saltzman DJ, Menger MD, et al. Systemic and subcutaneous microvascular Po2 dissociation during 4-h hemorrhagic shock in conscious hamsters. Am J Physiol 1996;270:H827–36.

19. Hurcombe SD, Welch BR, Williams JM, et al. Dark-field microscopy in the assessment of large colon microperfusion and mucosal injury in naturally occurring surgical disease of the equine large colon. Equine Vet J 2014;46:674–80.

20. Radcliffe RM, Divers TJ, Fletcher DJ, et al. Evaluation of L-lactate and cardiac troponin I in horses undergoing emergency abdominal surgery. J Vet Emerg Crit Care (San Antonio) 2012;22:313–9.

21. Salciccia A, Grulke S, de la Rebiere de Pouyade G, et al. Assessment of systemic inflammation by time-trends of blood granulocyte count and plasma myeloperoxidase and elastase concentrations following colic surgery in horses. J Vet Emerg Crit Care (San Antonio) 2016;26:541–8.

22. Dugdale AH, Barron KE, Miller AJ, et al. Effects of preoperative administration of hypertonic saline or pentastarch solution on hematologic variables and long-term survival of surgically managed horses with colic. J Am Vet Med Assoc 2015;246: 1104–11.

23. Classen DC, Evans RS, Pestotnik SL, et al. The timing of prophylactic administration of antibiotics and the risk of surgical-wound infection. N Engl J Med 1992; 326:281–6.
24. Dallap Schaer BL, Linton JK, Aceto H. Antimicrobial use in horses undergoing colic surgery. J Vet Intern Med 2012;26:1449–56.
25. Kito Y, Suzuki H. Effects of temperature on pacemaker potentials in the mouse small intestine. Pflugers Arch 2007;454:263–75.
26. Fintl C, Hudson NP, Handel I, et al. The effect of temperature changes on in vitro slow wave activity in the equine ileum. Equine Vet J 2016;48:218–23.
27. Guschlbauer M, Feige K, Geburek F, et al. Effects of in vivo lidocaine administration at the time of ischemia and reperfusion on in vitro contractility of equine jejunal smooth muscle. Am J Vet Res 2011;72:1449–55.
28. Guschlbauer M, Hoppe S, Geburek F, et al. In vitro effects of lidocaine on the contractility of equine jejunal smooth muscle challenged by ischaemia-reperfusion injury. Equine Vet J 2010;42:53–8.
29. Senior JM, Proudman CJ, Leuwer M, et al. Plasma endotoxin in horses presented to an equine referral hospital: correlation to selected clinical parameters and outcomes. Equine Vet J 2011;43:585–91.
30. Fogle J, Jacob M, Blikslager A, et al. Comparison of lipopolysaccharides and soluble CD14 measurement between clinically endotoxaemic and nonendotoxaemic horses. Equine Vet J 2017;49(2):155–9.
31. Moore JN, Vandenplas ML. Is it the systemic inflammatory response syndrome or endotoxemia in horses with colic? Vet Clin North Am Equine Pract 2014;30: 337–51, vii–viii.
32. Peiro JR, Barnabe PA, Cadioli FA, et al. Effects of lidocaine infusion during experimental endotoxemia in horses. J Vet Intern Med 2010;24:940–8.
33. Jacobs CC, Holcombe SJ, Cook VL, et al. Ethyl pyruvate diminishes the inflammatory response to lipopolysaccharide infusion in horses. Equine Vet J 2013; 45:333–9.
34. Bauquier JR, Tudor E, Bailey SR. Anti-inflammatory effects of four potential anti-endotoxaemic drugs assessed in vitro using equine whole blood assays. J Vet Pharmacol Ther 2015;38:290–6.
35. Morresey PR, Mackay RJ. Endotoxin-neutralizing activity of polymyxin B in blood after IV administration in horses. Am J Vet Res 2006;67:642–7.
36. Hassel DM, Smith PA, Nieto JE, et al. Di-tri-octahedral smectite for the prevention of post-operative diarrhea in equids with surgical disease of the large intestine: results of a randomized clinical trial. Vet J 2009;182:210–4.
37. Little D, Jones SL, Blikslager AT. Cyclooxygenase (COX) inhibitors and the intestine. J Vet Intern Med 2007;21:367–77.
38. Marshall JF, Blikslager AT. The effect of nonsteroidal anti-inflammatory drugs on the equine intestine. Equine Vet J Suppl 2011;(39):140–4.
39. Cook VL, Meyer CT, Campbell NB, et al. Effect of firocoxib or flunixin meglumine on recovery of ischemic-injured equine jejunum. Am J Vet Res 2009;70: 992–1000.
40. Little D, Brown SA, Campbell NB, et al. Effects of the cyclooxygenase inhibitor meloxicam on recovery of ischemia-injured equine jejunum. Am J Vet Res 2007;68:614–24.
41. Cook VL, Blikslager AT. The use of nonsteroidal anti-inflammatory drugs in critically ill horses. J Vet Emerg Crit Care (San Antonio) 2015;25:76–88.
42. Cox S, Villarino N, Sommardahl C, et al. Disposition of firocoxib in equine plasma after an oral loading dose and a multiple dose regimen. Vet J 2013;198:382–5.

43. Naylor RJ, Taylor AH, Knowles E, et al. Comparison of flunixin meglumine and me-loxicam for post-operative management of horses with strangulating small intes-tinal lesions. Equine Vet J 2014;46(4):427–34.
44. Lefebvre D, Hudson NP, Elce YA, et al. Clinical features and management of equine postoperative ileus (POI): Survey of Diplomates of the American Colleges of Veterinary Internal Medicine (ACVIM), Veterinary Surgeons (ACVS) and Veter-inary Emergency and Critical Care (ACVECC). Equine Vet J 2016;48(6):714–9.
45. Cook VL, Jones Shults J, McDowell M, et al. Attenuation of ischaemic injury in the equine jejunum by administration of systemic lidocaine. Equine Vet J 2008;40: 353–7.
46. Cook VL, Jones Shults J, McDowell MR, et al. Anti-inflammatory effects of intra-venously administered lidocaine hydrochloride on ischemia-injured jejunum in horses. Am J Vet Res 2009;70:1259–68.
47. Cook VL, Neuder LE, Blikslager AT, et al. The effect of lidocaine on in vitro adhe-sion and migration of equine neutrophils. Vet Immunol Immunopathol 2009;129: 137–42.
48. Little D, Tomlinson JE, Blikslager AT. Post operative neutrophilic inflammation in equine small intestine after manipulation and ischaemia. Equine Vet J 2005;37: 329–35.
49. Torfs S, Delesalle C, Dewulf J, et al. Risk factors for equine postoperative ileus and effectiveness of prophylactic lidocaine. J Vet Intern Med 2009;23:606–11.
50. Salem SE, Proudman CJ, Archer DC. Has intravenous lidocaine improved the outcome in horses following surgical management of small intestinal lesions in a UK hospital population? BMC Vet Res 2016;12:157.

Advances in Diagnostics and Treatments in Horses and Foals with Gastric and Duodenal Ulcers

Pilar Camacho-Luna, DVM[a], Benjamin Buchanan, DVM[b],
Frank M. Andrews, DVM, MS[a],*

KEYWORDS

- Horse • Equine • Gastric ulcer • Equine gastric ulcer syndrome • Diagnostics
- Therapeutics

KEY POINTS

- Equine gastric ulcer syndrome (EGUS) primarily describes ulceration in the terminal esophagus, nonglandular squamous mucosa, glandular mucosa of the stomach, and proximal duodenum.
- There are no pathognomonic clinical signs that indicate this diagnosis; however, clinical signs, fecal occult blood, urinary sucrose concentration, and response to treatment suggest EGUS, but the only definitive diagnosis is made with endoscopic examination of the stomach.
- Lesions in the squamous mucosa improve with altered management, dietary changes, and pharmacologic agents, whereas ulcers in glandular region for the most part are less likely to improve or are slow to improve.
- Omeprazole, a potent proton pump inhibitor, is currently the drug of choice for treatment and prevention of ulcers; however, many other pharmaceutical agents including antacids, H_2-receptor antagonists, sucralfate, and prostaglandin analogues have been used alone or with omeprazole to treat and prevent EGUS.

Disclosure Statement: The corresponding author, Dr F.M. Andrews, has received research funding from the LSU Foundation (Equine Fund), Merial Limited, and Purina Animal Nutrition. Dr F. M. Andrews is not an employee or a consultant for any company mentioned in this article.
[a] Equine Health Studies Program, Department of Veterinary Clinical Sciences, School of Veterinary Medicine, Louisiana State University, Skip Bertman Drive, Baton Rouge, LA 70803, USA;
[b] Brazos Valley Equine Hospital, 6999 HWY 6, Navasota, TX 77868, USA
* Corresponding author.
E-mail address: fandrews@lsu.edu

INTRODUCTION

Equine gastric ulcer syndrome (EGUS) is common in all breeds and ages of horses and foals. This article focuses on the current terminology for EGUS, etiologies and pathogenesis for lesions in the nonglandular and glandular stomach, diagnosis, and a comprehensive approach to the treatment and prevention of EGUS in adult horses and foals.

DEFINITION AND TERMINOLOGY

EGUS terminology was introduced in 1999[1] as an umbrella term to highlight the similarities to peptic ulcer disease in people[2] and described ulceration in the terminal esophagus, nonglandular stomach (squamous mucosa), glandular stomach, and proximal duodenum. A recent consensus statement reinforced this original umbrella terminology of EGUS (**Fig. 1**).[3]

Lesions in the nonglandular squamous mucosa (ESGD) are the result of increased exposure to aggressive factors, such as gastric acids (hydrochloric acid [HCl], volatile fatty acids, bile acids, and lactic acid) and pepsin **Table 1**.[4,5]

Equine glandular gastric disease (EGGD), lesions in the glandular mucosa, is emerging as an important disease.[3,6] HCl and a low stomach pH contribute to acid injury in the glandular mucosa. However, the mucosal defense mechanisms are likely compromised first, which allows backflow of HCl and organic acids into and between glandular cells, resulting in damage to the sodium pump **Table 1**.[7] Stress, infection with bacteria, nonsteroidal anti-inflammatory drugs (NSAIDs), and inhibition of secretion of protective prostaglandins are likely culprits.[6] Furthermore, observed lesions in the glandular stomach are frequently raised, with petechial hemorrhages and hyperemia, secondary to inflammation (**Fig. 2**). Such lesions might be an indication of inflammatory bowel disease and further evaluation of the gastrointestinal tract might be warranted, similar to Crohn disease in people affecting mucosa and deeper layers of the bowel wall and duodenum and leading to pyloric inflammation.[8]

PREVALENCE AND CLINICAL SIGNS
Adult Horses

The prevalence of ESGD varies from 40% to 90% in performance horses.[9] The prevalence of EGGD varies from 8% in thoroughbred racehorses in the United Kingdom to

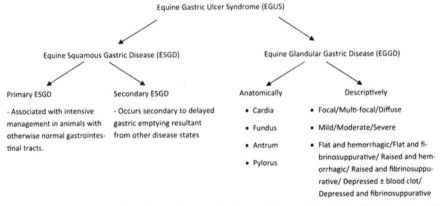

Fig. 1. Expanded terminology for equine gastric ulcer syndrome. (*From* Sykes BW, Hewetson M, Hepburn RJ, et al. European College of Equine Internal Medicine Consensus Statement—Equine Gastric Ulcer Syndrome in Adult Horses. J Vet Intern Med 2015;29:1289; with permission.)

Table 1
Physiologic factors affecting ulcer development

Aggressive Factors	Protective Factors: Nonglandular Mucosa	Protective Factors: Glandular Mucosa
Hydrochloric acid secretion	Epithelial restitution	Bicarbonate, mucus layer secretion
Organic acid production	Mucosal blood flow	Epithelial restitution
Pepsin conversion from pepsinogen		Mucosal blood flow
Duodenal reflux of bile acids		Prostaglandin E production

From Yuki N, Shimazaki T, Kushiro A, et al. Colonization of the stratified squamous epithelium of the nonsecreting area of horse stomach by lactobacilli. Appl Environ Microbiol 2000;66:5030–4; and Sykes BW, Sykes MK, Hallowell GD. Administration of trimethoprim-sulphadimidine does not improve healing of glandular gastric ulceration in horses receiving omeprazole: a randomized, blinded, clinical study. BMC Vet Res 2014;10:180; with permission.

63% of thoroughbred race horses in Australia. Based on an abattoir in the United Kingdom, ESGD and EGGD had high prevalence in domesticated horses (60.8% and 70.6%) compared with feral (22.2% and 29.6%) horses.[10] Some important risk factors for EGUS are age and gender; training; concurrent disease, such as impaction colic, colonic tympany, and intussusception; primary inflammatory bowel diseases, such as duodenitis-proximal jejunitis; diet; and the environment. The induction of ESGD with exercise, high-concentrate/low-roughage diets, fasting, transport, stall confinement, the administration of hypertonic electrolytes, and intermittent access to water can be rapid, occurring within 7 days in some studies and the risk of disease increasing with time in work.[9]

Clinical signs of ulcers are numerous and vague and include inappetence, poor body condition, weight loss, diarrhea, changes in behavior, and poor performance.[11–14] Colic is common in horses with EGUS. Other nonspecific signs include "pain or discomfort" when tightening the girth strap, and stereotypic or abnormal behavior, such as crib-biting, head nodding, stall wall kicking, stall pawing, wood chewing, flehmen, and stall weaving. In another study, there was no association between crib-biting/weaving and gastric ulceration.[14] Clinical signs of Equine Squamous Gastric Disease (ESGD) do not necessarily correlate with presence or severity of gastric ulcers.

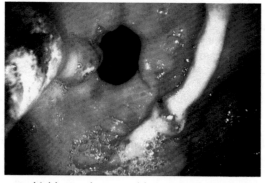

Fig. 2. Hyperemia, petechial hemorrhage, and hyperemia in the pyloric antrum, showing the typical lesions seen in the glandular region of the equine stomach.

Foals

The prevalence of EGUS in neonatal foals was estimated to be 25% to 50%.[15] Clinical signs in foal differ from those in adults. Classically, EGUS in foals has been divided into four clinical syndromes: (1) subclinical, (2) clinical, (3) perforating, and (4) gastric outflow obstruction secondary pyloric stricture.[16] The clinical signs of EGUS in foals with gastric outflow obstruction encompass those of gastroduodenal ulcer syndrome. Affected foals are often 2 to 6 months of age and typically shows signs of lethargy, colic, an unthrifty appearance, frequent recumbency, bruxism, ptyalism, frothing or drooling of milk from the mouth, interrupted nursing, tongue lolling, diarrhea (present or recent), and frequent rolling into dorsal recumbency.[17] Although clinical signs often do not necessarily correlate with a diagnosis of EGUS, they are used to suggest the diagnosis and recommend confirmation of lesions with gastroscopic examination. Typically, foals showing clinical signs of disease (eg, salivation, bruxism) have severe gastric lesions when present, but the clinical signs may also indicate other gastrointestinal disease, such as small intestinal intussusceptions, small intestinal volvulus, peritonitis, impaction, diaphragmatic hernia, enterocolitis, and gastric outflow obstruction.[17] Previous and concurrent diarrhea were reported in foals with endoscopic-confirmed EGUS. Recently the use of antiulcer medications was shown to increase the odds ($\times 2$) of diarrhea in hospitalized foals, but did not increase the risk of diarrhea caused by *Clostridium* spp.[18]

DIAGNOSIS

The definitive diagnosis of EGUS is based on endoscopic evidence of gastric erosion, ulceration, or other lesions. In addition, a presumptive diagnosis of EGUS is made based on history, clinical signs, and response to treatment. Currently, there are no hematologic or biochemical markers to diagnose EGUS. Because of the lack of additional methods of laboratory diagnosis, in situations where ulcers are strongly suspected but gastroscopy is not available, it may be worthwhile to start empiric treatment and observe for resolution of clinical signs. If the horse does not respond to treatment, referral to a facility with a gastroscope is indicated.

The fecal occult blood test (Succeed FBT, Freedom Health LLC, Lexington, KY) currently on the market has demonstrated high specificity and low sensitivity and high false-negative results for diagnosis of EGUS.[19,20] Thus, its use to diagnose EGUS is limited, but might be helpful to diagnose and document healing in horses with hindgut disease, such as colitis.

Gastroscopy is the only method currently available to obtain a definitive diagnosis of gastric ulcers. Proper standing gastroscopy requires a 3-m endoscope to adequately visualize the nonglandular and glandular stomach, pylorus, and proximal duodenum in most adult horses. Recently the European College of Equine Internal Medicine consensus statement recommended the use of a common scoring system modified from the original US omeprazole trials because it is easy to use and accurate.[3] Ulcers in the terminal esophagus may indicate a gastric outflow obstruction caused by pyloric ulceration or stenosis (**Fig. 3**). Hyperkeratosis (**Fig. 4**) and hyperemia (**Figs. 5**) should also be recorded along with the ulcer score. The exact cause of hyperkeratosis is unknown but it is not thought to be proliferation or thickening of the nonglandular mucosa secondary to acid exposure and does not require treatment. In addition, hyperkeratosis may be seen around healing ulcers as the first stage of epithelial repair. In contrast, hyperemia, primarily seen in the glandular stomach, might be associated with inflammation. In people, hyperemia is almost always associated with inflammatory changes caused by *Helicobacter* spp; however, hyperemia in the glandular mucosa in adult

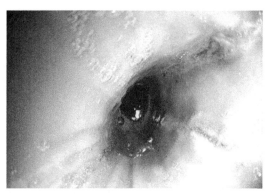

Fig. 3. Linear ulcerations in the terminal esophagus of a pony with a gastric outflow obstruction secondary to pyloric stenosis.

horses and foals has not been extensively evaluated. Most glandular lesions in adult horses do not seem to have true ulcer characteristics (depressed ulcer bed), but may be raised with petechial hemorrhages (see **Fig. 2**). To establish a diagnosis for such lesions, four biopsies should be taken from the abnormal areas and biopsies of the glandular mucosa yield the best specimens for diagnosis.[21] Squamous mucosal biopsies are usually superficial and do not yield diagnostic samples in most specimens.

In foals, endoscopy and ultrasound are the most important diagnostic tools for confirming mucosal ulcers and visually observing gastric and duodenal motility, respectively. Contrast radiography of the stomach following a barium swallow has also been used to confirm delayed gastric emptying (**Fig. 6**).[22]

TREATMENT OF EQUINE GASTRIC ULCER SYNDROME
Environmental, Nutritional, and Dietary Management

Without alterations in management or initiation of preventative therapy, squamous ulcers quickly return if horses are maintained in training.[23] Reducing exercise intensity, increasing pasture turnout, and amending dietary risk factors might help decrease ulcer severity and the risk of recurrence in squamous ulcers, but it is unknown if this

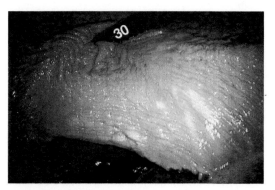

Fig. 4. Hyperkeratosis in the nonglandular mucosa, lesser curvature. Note the endoscope dorsally exiting the terminal esophagus.

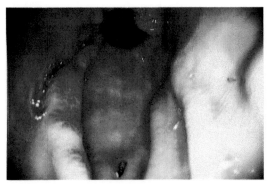

Fig. 5. Hyperemia without ulceration in the glandular mucosa, pyloric antrum. Note the opening to the duodenum.

prevents recurrence of glandular ulcers. The following recommendations are primarily for squamous ulcers, but might have a positive effect on glandular ulcers[9]: (1) modification of exercise intensity and duration, (2) increase pasture turnout, (3) eliminate bolus feeding and increase forage/fiber intake, and (4) reduce the intake of nonstructural carbohydrate.

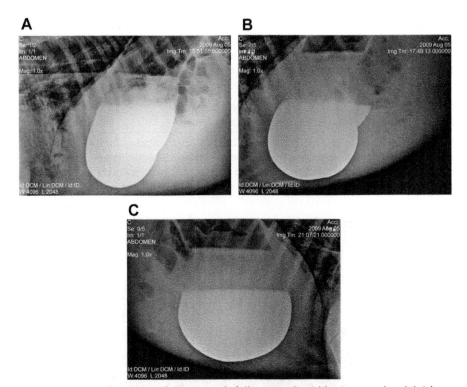

Fig. 6. Contrast radiography of the stomach following a liquid barium meal at (*A*) 0 hour, (*B*) 2 hours, and (*C*) 6 hours showing delayed gastric emptying caused by pyloric stenosis. Typical gastric emptying of a liquid meal is 30 to 45 minutes.

Antibiotics Versus Probiotics Versus Prebiotics

Helicobacter pylori and other *Helicobacter* species have not been shown to cause squamous or glandular ulcers in horses, although *Helicobacter* DNA has been isolated from the squamous and glandular mucosa of horses.[24] Instead, other resident, acid-tolerant bacteria (*Escherichia coli, Lactobacillus,* and *Streptococcus*) are suspected to contribute to the worsening of squamous ulcers.[25] A large population of these bacteria were isolated from the gastric contents of horses fed various diets in that study. In a study evaluating horses with spontaneously occurring squamous ulcers, an antibiotic (trimethoprim sulphadimidine) or a probiotic preparation containing *Lactobacillus agilis, Lactobacillus salivarius, Lactobacillus equi, Streptococcus equinus,* and *Streptococcus bovis* administered orally decreased ulcer number and severity compared with untreated control subjects.[25] These data suggest that resident stomach bacteria are important in maintenance and progression of squamous ulcers in horses. In addition, administration of probiotics containing *Lactobacillus* spp might protect the squamous mucosa from ulcer formation by colonization of the mucosa.[26] Antibiotic treatment may be indicated in horses with chronic nonresponsive squamous ulcers. However, once-daily administration of trimethoprim-sulphadimidine did not improve healing of glandular gastric ulceration in horses receiving omeprazole.[27] Antibiotics should be used responsibly and only when acid-suppressive therapy alone is not effective.

A recent short-term (90-day treatment) study evaluating the effect of a prebiotic dietary supplement (Succeed Digestive Conditioning System, Freedom Health, LLC, Aurora, OH) showed the product was noninferior (similar efficacy) to 4 mg/kg omeprazole administered daily in the proportion of horses with complete resolution of squamous ulceration.[28] However, in that study, 10 of 21 horses in the trial on omeprazole had at least one period of forced withdrawal because of racing rules from treatment at some point during the trial and it likely reduced efficacy of omeprazole at Day 90. Further research is needed to determine the efficacy of prebiotics or probiotics on stomach health and these products should not be used to treat ulcers, but rather as an adjunct therapy to maintain gastrointestinal health in horses with EGUS.

PHARMACOLOGIC THERAPY

Only approximately 4% to 6% of nonglandular ulcers heal spontaneously; to achieve significant healing, most horses need pharmacologic therapy, especially when they remain in athletic training.[23]

Nonglandular ulcers respond well to agents that increase gastric juice pH. However, the efficacy of pharmaceutical agents on EGGD has not been thoroughly studied; treatment of EGGD often follows the same principles as for ESGD, but a longer treatment period with omeprazole might be required.[3]

Proton Pump Inhibitors

Omeprazole paste (GastroGard paste, Merial Limited, Duluth, GA) is registered in several countries for treatment and prevention of recurrence of EGUS.[23] However, other pharmaceutical agents and their doses are listed in **Table 2**.[9]

Omeprazole decreases gastric acid secretion by blocking hydrogen-potassium-ATPase in the secretory membrane of parietal cells. This enzyme catalyzes the exchange of hydrogen ions for potassium ions in the final step of hydrochloric acid production by parietal cells. Omeprazole is 10 times more potent than ranitidine

Table 2
Commonly used therapeutic agents for treatment and prevention of gastric ulcers in horses and foals

Drug	Dose (mg/kg)	Dosing Interval (h)	Route of Administration
Ranitidine	6.6	q 6–8	PO
Ranitidine	1.5	q 6	IV, IM
Omeprazole	4 (treatment)	q 24	PO
Omeprazole	1–2 (prevention)	q 24	PO
Omeprazole	0.5–1.0	q 24	IV
Esomeprazole	1.0 mg/kg	q 24	IV
Esomeprazole	1.0–2.0 mg/kg	q 24	PO
Pantoprazole	1.0–1.5	q 24	IV or PO
Sucralfate	12–20	q 8	PO
Al- or Mg hydroxide	0.5 mL/kg	q 4–6	PO
Misoprostol, prostaglandin analogues	1–5 μg	q 8–12	PO

Abbreviations: IM, intramuscular; IV, intravenous.
From Buchanan BR, Andrews FM. Treatment and prevention of equine gastric ulcer syndrome. Vet Clin Equine 2003;19:582; with permission.

on an equimolar basis.[29] Several reports have suggested that depending on the formulation, a lower dose of omeprazole (1.0 mg/kg, orally every 24 hours) might be effective if administered before exercise and following a brief fast.[30] In that study fewer glandular ulcers healed (36%), when compared with squamous ulcers (78%). The results demonstrated differences in healing rates depending on ulcer location.

In addition, the bioavailability of omeprazole is affected by formulation and feeding, because the omeprazole powder is acid labile and inactivated by stomach acid. Although only omeprazole paste formulation (GastroGard, Merial Limited) is Food and Drug Administration (FDA)-approved in the United States, several formulations are available over the counter and from compounding pharmacies. Recently the bioavailability of several formulations was tested in horses and an enteric-coated omeprazole formulation (21.5% [9.0–27.7]) was approximately two times higher than a plain paste formulation of omeprazole (10.1% [7.7–13.3]).[31] In addition, feeding had minimal effect on the bioavailability of either formulation. The bioavailability of the FDA-approved omeprazole paste was reported to be 12% to 16% and was higher (16%) in fasted horses. It should be noted that the area under the curve for omeprazole concentration was higher in the enteric-coated granule formulation, when compared with the plain paste formulation in that study.[31] Omeprazole paste has been shown to have a wide safety margin and is effective in foals 3 months old and mature horses.[32]

Recent investigations have shown a reduced efficacy in omeprazole-treated horses with EGGD, when compared with ESGD. Only 36% of glandular ulcers healed when treated with omeprazole (4 mg/kg, orally every 24 hours) compared with a 78% healing rate in horses with diagnosed ESGD.[30] The reason for this is not known, but is likely a reflection of the different pathogenesis causing EGGD, compared with ESGD. As such glandular ulcers deserve to be considered as a related but distinct disease to the traditional ESGD ulcers.

Esomeprazole, the S-enantiomer of omeprazole, provides better gastric acid control and decreases interindividual variability in gastric juice pH in people, when compared with omeprazole.[33] The improved efficacy of esomeprazole is likely caused by a lower plasma clearance and larger area under curve for plasma concentration-time when compared with omeprazole. Higher plasma concentrations result in greater drug availability to inhibit parietal cell HCl secretion. One study showed that intravenous (IV) administration of esomeprazole to horses for 14 days significantly increased gastric juice pH.[34] In addition, oral administration of esomeprazole (Nexium, AstraZeneca Pharmaceuticals LP, Wilmington, DE; 40 mg or 80 mg, orally every 24 hours) controlled pH levels of gastric secretions in thoroughbreds.[35] The results corroborated the efficacy of esomeprazole magnesium in the control of gastric pH at both doses tested, with 100% of the mean pH being greater than 5 and no statistical difference was noted between the two doses tested.

Pantoprazole, another proton pump inhibitor, has been evaluated in foals. Pantoprazole was administered IV (1.5 mg/kg) and enterally through a nasogastric tube (1.5 mg/kg, Body Weight [BWT]) to neonatal foals.[36] Gastric juice pH increased significantly after IV and intragastric administration. Pantoprazole could be used IV in foals with pyloric outflow obstruction, especially because IV administration of ranitidine has shown inconsistent effects on increasing gastric juice pH. However, intragastric administration of pantoprazole resulted in a lower bioavailability, when compared with oral administration of omeprazole, so a higher dose should be used if administered orally in foals.

Histamine Type 2 Receptor Blockers

Histamine type-2 receptor antagonists suppress HCl secretion by reversibly binding and competitively inhibiting the parietal cell H_2 receptors. Ranitidine and cimetidine are two drugs of this type used in the horse. Ranitidine is available in tablet, syrup, suspension, and injectable forms. Unfortunately, ranitidine requires three times daily oral administration and longer treatment duration (45–60 days), compared with omeprazole (28 days) to achieve similar healing.[9] Ranitidine was less effective than omeprazole in healing gastric ulcers in race horses.[37] Cimetidine, however, does not seem to be effective in treatment of EGUS and is not recommended.

Coating Agents

Sucralfate binds to stomach ulcers and promotes healing. Sucralfate is an aluminum complex sulfated polysaccharide (α-D-glucopyranoside, β-Dfructofuranosyl-, octakis-[hydrogen sulfate]), in combination with octasulfate and aluminum hydroxide. Its mechanism of action involves adherence to ulcerated mucosa, forming a proteinaceous bandage, and stimulating prostaglandin E_1 synthesis and mucus secretion. Sucralfate also inactivates pepsin and adsorbs bile acids. Recently, sucralfate (12 mg/kg, orally every 8 hours) alone or combined with omeprazole was recommended to treat glandular ulcers, but was not as effective as misoprostol alone.[3,5,38]

Equine sucralfate malate paste (Mucosalfate, brand of Orafate, Mueller Medical International LLC, Storrs, CT) was approved in 2013 by the FDA to treat oral and esophageal ulcerations and erosions, equine stomatitis, and periogingival inflammation.[39] The product is a polymerized, cross-linked 10% sucralfate paste. It also contains xanthan gum, calcium sulfate, purified water, calcium carbonate, methyl parabens, propyl parabens, malate, and sodium saccharin in a strawberry flavor. Water containing calcium chelated malic acid is added to sucralfate powder, thereby converting sucralfate granules into a polymerized paste. Mucosalfate forms a protective layer over the oral mucosa by adhering to the mucosal surface, which allows it to protect against further irritation and relieve pain. The paste may be used in the management of a variety of oral and esophageal lesions in horses, including those caused by periodontal and gingival inflammation, tooth extractions, traumatic wounds, and wounds associated with oral surgery.[40] The authors have used this product to successfully treat esophageal and colonic ulcers. It might also be effective, when administered with omeprazole, to treat EGGD; however, data are lacking.

Porcine hydrolyzed collagen (HC; Hydro-P Premium, Sonac, A Darling Ingredient Company, Son, The Netherlands) was recently evaluated in stall-confined horses treated with omeprazole and undergoing intermittent feeding. The HC (45 g) was mixed with sweet feed twice daily for 56 days in a two-period crossover study.[41] Mean gastric juice pH was higher in the HC-treated horses, while the horses were on omeprazole treatment. In addition, HC-treated horses resulted in fewer ulcers at each gastroscopic examination and a significant effect on ulcer scores was seen on Day 56 of treatment.

Antacids

Calcium carbonate is commonly used as an antacid in people. In in vitro studies, exposure of nonglandular mucosa to calcium carbonate resulted in recovery of tissue exposed to stomach acid. In addition, dietary studies feeding alfalfa hay, which contains a high concentration of calcium carbonate and protein, improved nonglandular gastric ulcer scores and increased gastric juice pH in stall-confined horses and horse that were exercising.[42,43]

Synthetic Prostaglandins

The synthetic prostaglandin E_2 analogue, misoprostol, has been recommended to treat EGUS.[3,9] Misoprostol is a methylester analogue of prostaglandin, and it showed a time-dependent increase in the basal gastric pH in horses Misoprostol enhances mucosal protection by stimulating mucus and bicarbonate production, and may aid in the treatment and prevention of EGGD.[44]

In addition to increasing mucus and bicarbonate secretion, a recent report showed that misoprostol significantly inhibited inflammatory mediators (tumor necrosis factor-α, interleukin-1b, and interleukin-6 and superoxide) produced ex vivo from equine leukocytes exposed to lipolysaccarhide.[45] This study showed that misoprostol has anti-inflammatory effects that might be effective in treating EGGD, because many lesions in the glandular mucosa might be inflammatory. In a more recent study, misoprostol (5 μg/kg, orally every 12 hours) was found to be superior to combined omeprazole (4 mg/kg, orally every 24 hours) and sucralfate (12 mg/kg, orally every 12 hours) therapy in horses with EGGD.[38] Misoprostol might cause diarrhea and/or colic signs and should not be used in pregnant mares, because it might induce parturition and termination of the pregnancy.

Motility Stimulants

Bethanechol is a synthetic muscarinic cholinergic agent that is not degraded by acetylcholinesterases. Bethanechol (0.25 mg/kg, IV) and erythromycin lactobionate (0.1 and 1 mg/kg IV) increased solid-phase gastric emptying in horses.[46] No significant adverse effects were observed in healthy horses; however, other forms of erythromycin can cause fatal colitis in adult horses at antimicrobial doses. The only side effect of bethanechol administration was increased salivation. Authors have recommended a dose of 0.025 to 0.03 mg/kg subcutaneously every 3 to 4 hours, followed by oral

Table 3
Treatment recommendations for equine squamous gastric disease

Primary Recommendation	Secondary Recommendation
Omeprazole	Omeprazole
Buffered formulations, 4 mg/kg PO, q 24 h; or	Buffered formulation, 2 mg/kg PO q 24 h
Enteric-coated granule formulations, 1 mg/kg PO q 24 h; or	Or
	Ranitidine, 6.6 mg/kg PO q 8 h
Plain formulations, 4 mg/kg PO q 24 h	
Treatment duration, 3 wk	
Control gastroscopy before the discontinuation of treatment	

maintenance therapy at 0.3 to 0.45 mg/kg three to four times daily. Prokinetics should not be used in horses with gastrointestinal obstructions, because it is possible that gastroduodenal reflux may worsen after treatment in patients with proximal small intestinal obstructions.

Treatment and Prevention Recommendations

A summary of treatment recommendations for equine squamous ESGD and EGGD is found in **Tables 3** and **4**. Given the recent evidence of cyclooxygenase-2 activity in glandular tissue and the oxidative stress induced by NSAIDs in glandular tissues, avoidance of NSAIDs including cyclooxygenase-2-selective inhibitors in horses at risk for EGGD should be considered.[47]

As a reminder, compounded medications from bulk powders is currently illegal in the United States, according to the FDA, especially when there is an approved drug available and compounded omeprazole has been shown to be less efficacious than the FDA-approved omeprazole paste.[48]

For the treatment and prevention of EGUS in foals, clinicians should follow similar principles as for adult horses. However, prophylactic treatment of hospitalized neonatal foals could increase the risk of diarrhea.[18] A multicenter retrospective study including 1710 foals ($\leq$10 days of age) showed that the use of antiulcer medications, including sucralfate, increased the odds of in-hospital diarrhea by $\times$2, relative to those foals who received no antiulcer medications. Thus, use of antiulcer medications in hospitalized neonatal foals should be carefully evaluated on an individual basis.

Table 4
Treatment recommendation for equine glandular gastric disease

Primary Recommendation	Secondary Recommendation
Omeprazole	Omeprazole
Buffered formulations, 4 mg/kg PO q 24 h; or	Buffered formulations, 2 mg/kg PO q 24 h
Enteric-coated granule formulations, 1 mg/kg PO q 24 h; or	
Plain formulations, 4 mg/kg PO q 24 h	
Plus	Plus
Sucralfate, 12 mg/kg PO q 12 h	Sucralfate, 12 mg/kg PO q 12 h
	Or
	Specific nutraceutical with published efficacy
Treatment duration, 4 wk (minimum of 8 wk before additional adjunctives are considered)	
Control gastroscopy before the discontinuation of therapy	

SUMMARY

Currently, diagnosis of EGUS is based on endoscopic visualization of ulcers and omeprazole is accepted globally as the best pharmacologic therapy. A recent publication summarized the important nutritional and dietary recommendations to lessen severity and prevent EGUS.[49]

1. Keep the horse eating by providing a minimum of 1 to 1.5 kg/100 kg body weight of long-stem high-quality forage (hay) free-choice throughout the day and night.
2. Feed alfalfa hay or a mixture alfalfa hay to help buffer stomach acid.
3. Feed grain and concentrates sparingly. Give no more than 0.5 kg/100 kg body weight of grain or grain mixes, such as "sweet feed," and do not feed grain meals less than 6 hours apart.
4. Try corn oil or other dietary supplements, but feed hypertonic electrolyte pastes or supplements after exercise with a grain meal.
5. Consider therapeutic or preventative doses of effective pharmacologic agents in horses that are performing high-intensity exercise, traveling, or in a high-stress situation. This is especially important in horses with chronic arthritis and one should consider the following:
   A. Choose NSAIDs that have minimal effects on the gastrointestinal tract, such as firocoxib and ketoprofen.
   B. Doses of NSAIDs should be used at the minimal dose that effectively controls pain.
   C. If NSAIDs are used, then administering antiulcer medications at preventative or treatment doses should be considered.

REFERENCES

1. Andrews FM, Bernard W, Byars D, et al. Recommendation for the diagnosis and treatment of equine gastric ulcer syndrome (EGUS). Equine Vet Educ 1999;11: 262–72.
2. Malfertheiner P, Chan FFKL, McColl KEL, et al. Peptic-ulcer disease. Lancet 2009;374:1449–61.
3. Sykes BW, Hutson M, Hepburn RJ, et al. European College of Equine Internal Medicine Consensus Statement: equine gastric ulcer syndrome in adult horse. J Vet Intern Med 2015;29:1288–99.
4. Andrews FM, Buchanan BR, Smith SH, et al. In vitro effects of hydrochloric acid and various concentrations of acetic, propionic, butyric, or valeric acids on bioelectric properties of equine gastric squamous mucosa. Am J Vet Res 2006; 67(11):1873–82.
5. Peretich AL, Abbott LL, Andrews FM, et al. Age-dependent regulation of sodium-potassium adenosinetriphosphatase and sodium-hydrogen exchanger mRNAs in equine nonglandular mucosa. Am J Vet Res 2009;70:1124–8.
6. Skyes BW, Jokisalo JM. Rethinking equine gastric ulcer syndrome: part 3-equine glandular gastric ulcer syndrome (EGGUS). Equine Vet Educ 2015;27:372–5.
7. Argenzio RA, Eisemann J. Mechanisms of acid injury in porcine gastroesophageal mucosa. Am J Vet Res 1996;57:564–73.
8. Kelly SM, Hunter JO. Endoscopic balloon dilatation of duodenal strictures in Crohn's disease. Postgrad Med J 1995;71:623–4.
9. Buchanan BR, Andrews FM. Treatment and prevention of equine gastric ulcer syndrome. Vet Clin Equine 2003;19:575–97.

10. Ward S, Sykes BW, Brown H, et al. A comparison of the prevalence of gastric ulceration in feral and domesticated horses in the UK. Equine Vet Educ 2015;57:655–7.
11. Franklin SH, Brazil TJ, Allen KJ. Poor performance associated with equine gastric ulceration syndrome in four thoroughbred racehorses. Equine Vet Educ 2008;20:119–24.
12. Nieto JE, Synder JR, Vatistas NJ, et al. Effect of gastric ulceration on physiologic responses to exercise in horses. Am J Vet Res 2009;70:787–95.
13. Vatistas NJ, Snyder JR, Carlson G, et al. Cross-sectional study of gastric ulcers of the squamous mucosa in thoroughbred racehorses. Equine Vet J 1999;29(Suppl):40–4.
14. Wickens C, McCall CA, Bursian S, et al. Assessment of gastric ulceration and gastrin response in horses with history of crib-biting. J Equine Vet Sci 2013;33:739–45.
15. Wilson JH. Gastric and duodenal ulcers in foals: a retrospective study. In: Proceedings of the Second Equine Colic Research Symposium. Athens (GA): Georgia Center for Continuing Education; Oct 1–3, 1986. p. 126–9.
16. Andrews FM, Nadeau JA. Clinical syndromes of gastric ulceration in foals and mature horses. Equine Vet J Suppl 1999;(29):30–3.
17. Murray MJ, Murray CM, Sweeney HJ, et al. Prevalence of gastric lesions in foals without signs of gastric disease: an endoscopic survey. Equine Vet J 1990;22:6–8.
18. Furr M, Cohen ND, Axon JE, et al. Treatment with histamine-type 2 receptor antagonists and omeprazole increase the risk of diarrhea in neonatal foals treated in intensive care units. Equine Vet J Suppl 2012;(41):80–6.
19. Pellegrini FL. Results of a large–scale necroscopic study of equine colonic ulcers. J Equine Vet Sci 2005;25:113–7.
20. Andrews FM, Camacho-Luna P, Loftin PG, et al. Effect of a pelleted supplement fed during and after omeprazole treatment on non-glandular gastric ulcer scores and gastric juice pH in horses. Equine Vet Educ 2015;28:196–202.
21. Murray MJ, Hepburn RJ, Sullins KE. Preliminary study of use of a polypectomy snare to obtain large samples of the equine gastric antrum by endoscopy. Equine Vet J 2004;36:76–8.
22. Campbell ML, Ackerman N, Peyton LC. Radiographic gastrointestinal anatomy of the foal. Vet Radiol Ultrasound 1984;25:194–204.
23. Andrews FM, Sifferman RL, Bernard W, et al. Efficacy of omeprazole paste in the treatment and prevention of gastric ulcers in horses. Equine Vet J Suppl 1999;(29):81–6.
24. Contreras M, Morales A, Garcia-Amado MA, et al. Detection of *Helicobacter*-like DNA in the gastric mucosa of thoroughbred horses. Lett Appl Microbiol 2007;45:553–7.
25. Al Jassim RAM, McGowan T, Andrews FM, et al. Role of bacteria and lactic acid in the pathogenesis of gastric ulceration. In: Rural industries research and development corporation final report. Brisbane (Australia): 2008. p. 1–26.
26. Yuki N, Shimazaki T, Kushiro A, et al. Colonization of the stratified squamous epithelium of the nonsecreting area of horse stomach by lactobacilli. Appl Environ Microbiol 2000;66:5030–4.
27. Sykes BW, Sykes MK, Hallowell GD. Administration of trimethoprim-sulphadimidine does not improve healing of glandular gastric ulceration in horses receiving omeprazole: a randomized, blinded, clinical study. BMC Vet Res 2014;10:180.
28. Kerybyson NC, Knottenbelt DK, Carslake HB, et al. A comparison between omeprazole and a dietary supplement for the management of squamous gastric ulceration in horses. J Equine Vet Sci 2016;40:94–101.

29. Walt RP, Gomes WD, Wood EC, et al. Effect of daily oral omeprazole on 24 hour intragastric acidity. Br Med J (Clin Res Ed) 1983;287:12–20.

30. Sykes BW, Sykes KM, Hallowell GD. A comparison of three doses of omeprazole in the treatment of equine gastric ulcer syndrome: a blinded, randomized, dose-response clinical trial. Equine Vet J 2015;47:285–90.

31. Sykes BW, Underwood C, McGowan CM, et al. Pharmacokinetics of intravenous, plain oral and enteric-coated oral omeprazole in the horse. J Vet Pharmacol Ther 2015;38:130–6.

32. Plue RE. Safety of omeprazole paste in foals and mature horses. Equine Vet J 1999;31(Suppl 29):63–6.

33. Scott LJ, Mallarkey G, Sharpe M. Esomeprazole: a review of its use in the management of acid-related disorders. Drugs 2002;62:1503–38.

34. Videla R, Sommardahl CS, Elliott SB, et al. Effects of intravenously administration esomeprazole sodium on gastric juice pH in adult female horses. J Vet Intern Med 2011;25:558–62.

35. Pereira MC, Levy FL, Valadão CAA, et al. Preliminary study of the gastric acidity in thoroughbred horses at rest after enteral administration of esomeprazole magnesium (nexium). J Equine Vet Sci 2009;29:791–4.

36. Ryan CA, Sanchez LC, Giguère S, et al. Pharmacokinetics and pharmacodynamics of pantoprazole in clinically normal neonatal foals. Equine Vet J 2005;4:336–41.

37. Lester GD, Smith RL, Robertson ID. Effects of treatment with omeprazole or ranitidine on gastric squamous ulceration in racing thoroughbreds. J Am Vet Med Assoc 2005;227:1636–9.

38. Georgina V, Bowen M, Nicholls V, et al. Misoprostol is superior to combined omeprazole and sucralfate for healing glandular gastric lesions in horses with clinical disease. In Proceedings of the ACVIM Forum. Denver, CO, June 9–11, 2016, p. E25.

39. Equine Mucosalfate™ (Brand of Orafate™) Prescribing Information FDA 510k 123904 – Cleared August 2013. Sterling Foster Animal Health (A Mueller Medical International, LLC Company).

40. McCollough RW. Expedited management of ulcer, colic and diarrhea in 209 horses: an open-labeled observational study of a potency-enhanced sucralfate-like elm phyto-saccharide. J Vet Med Anim Health Vol 2013;5:32–40.

41. Keowen ML, Camacho-Luna P, Micheau L, et al. Effects of collagen hydrolysates on equine gastric ulcer scores and gastric juice pH. J Vet Int Med 2016;30(4):1512.

42. Lybbert T, Gibbs P, Cohen N, et al. Feeding alfalfa hay to exercising horses reduces the severity of gastric squamous mucosal ulceration. In: Proceedings of the 53rd Annual Convention of the American Association of Equine Practitioners. Orlando, Florida, December 1-5, 2007. p. 525–6.

43. Nadeau JA, Andrews FM, Mathew AG, et al. Evaluation of diet as a cause of gastric ulcers in horses. Am J Vet Res 2000;61:784–90.

44. Medina SR, Reyes GG, Mateos GE. Prevention of gastroduodenal injury induced by NSAIDs with low-dose misoprostol. Proc West Pharmacol Soc 1998;42:33–4.

45. Medlin E, Jones S. Investigation of misoprostol as a novel anti-inflammatory in equine leukocytes. ACVIM Forum, June 7-10 Denver, CO. J Vet Intern Med Forum 2016;30:1520.

46. Ringger NC, Lester GD, Neuwirth L, et al. Effect of bethanechol or erythromycin on gastric emptying in horses. Am J Vet Res 1996;57:1771–5.

47. Martínez Aranzales JR, Cândido de Andrade BS, Silveira Alves GE. Orally administered phenylbutazone causes oxidative stress in the equine gastric mucosa. J Vet Pharmacol Ther 2015;38:257–64.
48. Merritt AM, Sanchez LC, Burrow JA, et al. Effect of GastroGard and three compounded oral omeprazole preparations on 24 h intragastric pH in gastrically cannulated mature horses. Equine Vet J 2003;35:691–5.
49. Andrews FM, Larson C, Harris P. Nutritional management of gastric ulceration. Equine Vet Educ 2017;29:45–55.

Equine Dysautonomia

Bruce C. McGorum, BSc, BVM&S, PhD, CEIM, FRCVS*,
R. Scott Pirie, BVM&S, PhD, CEIM, CEP, MRCVS

KEYWORDS

- Grass sickness • Dysautonomia • Ileus • Chromatolysis • Enteric nervous system

KEY POINTS

- Despite the adopted nomenclature, equine dysautonomia (ED; also known as equine grass sickness) is a multisystem neuropathy. Although the clinical phenotype is largely reflective of autonomic (including enteric) nervous system dysfunction, neuronal degeneration occurs at other nonautonomic neuroanatomic locations.
- ED primarily affects grazing equids, and several other disease-associated risk factors have been identified.
- The cause remains undetermined, although the currently favored etiologic hypotheses include *Clostridium botulinum* toxicoinfection and/or mycotoxicosis.
- Although the disease phenotype is subclassified as acute (severe), subacute (moderate), and chronic (mild), these represent different categories within a continuum of disease severities.
- The antemortem diagnostic approach relies on consideration of disease-associated risk factors, the clinical presentation of the patients, exclusion of other differential diagnoses, the adoption of appropriate ancillary diagnostic techniques, and, on occasion, histopathologic confirmation of enteric neuronal pathology.

INTRODUCTION

Equine dysautonomia (ED; also known as equine grass sickness) is a polyneuropathy affecting both the central and peripheral nervous systems of, almost exclusively, grazing horses. Following the original report of ED in 1907,[1] it has subsequently been recognized throughout most of Northern Europe.[2–11] Suspected cases have also been reported in the Falkland Islands[12] and Australia.[13] Although North America has largely been considered free of the disease, ED was recently described in a mule in the United States.[14] A clinically and pathologically identical disease, Mal Seco, is well recognized in South America.[15–18]

Despite the reported widespread neuroanatomical distribution of degenerative neuronal lesions in ED, the autonomic nervous system (ANS) and enteric nervous

The Dick Vet Equine Hospital, Royal (Dick) School of Veterinary Studies, University of Edinburgh, Easter Bush Campus, Easter Bush, Roslin, Midlothian EH25 9RG, GBR
* Corresponding author.
E-mail address: bruce.mcgorum@ed.ac.uk

Vet Clin Equine 34 (2018) 113–125
https://doi.org/10.1016/j.cveq.2017.11.010
0749-0739/18/© 2017 Elsevier Inc. All rights reserved.

system (ENS) remain the most consistently and severely affected.[19] The spectrum of clinical signs, which define ED largely but not exclusively, reflects involvement of the ANS and ENS. The severity of disease and gross pathologic findings can largely be attributed to the extent of enteric neuronal loss (see *physical examination findings* and *pathologic findings*).

Despite extensive research efforts over the past century, the cause of ED remains elusive. Current research efforts are primarily focused on the potential role of either *Clostridium botulinum* neurotoxins (via toxicoinfection)[20–22] or ingested pasture-derived mycotoxins.[23,24] The *C botulinum* hypothesis was extensively investigated during the 1920s[25] and has recently received renewed interest. **Table 1** summarizes the factors that either support or refute the involvement of *C botulinum* in ED. In addition to the key association with grazing, the hypothesized role of pasture-derived mycotoxins in ED is largely justified by the seasonality of the disease[33,34] and the geographic and temporal clustering of cases,[35] which likely reflect climatic influences on etiologic agent exposure.[33,36]

PATIENT HISTORY

Consideration of the history of both the patients and the premises is beneficial in ED diagnosis. Appropriate questioning of the owner will allow the clinician to ascertain which of the published risk factors apply to the case and consider the diagnostic value of any relevant associations. A summary of the various published horse-, premise-, management-, and climate-level factors associated with either an increased or decreased risk of ED occurrence, or recurrence on a previously affected premise, is presented in **Table 2**. It is worth noting that, despite a general agreement between studies, occasional inconsistencies exist with regard to some of these reported associations.

As well as carefully considering the applicability of some of the risk factors in each case, a careful clinical history should also be obtained. Typically, severe (acute) cases of ED will have a sudden onset, with little prior indication of impending disease. In contrast, mild (chronic) cases will typically have an insidious onset, whereby

Table 1
Factors that support and refute involvement of *Clostridium botulinum* in equine dysautonomia

Supportive Factors	Refutative Factors
• Reportedly successful historic botulinum vaccine trial (1922 and 1923)[25]	• Disease phenotypic differences between ED and neuroparalytic botulism[24]
• Significantly greater prevalence of intestinal *C botulinum* bacteria and/or toxin in patients with ED vs control animals[20–22]	• Greater prevalence of other (non–*C botulinum*) clostridial species in intestinal tract of patients with ED vs controls (possibly reflecting generalized clostridial overgrowth)[30,31]
• Risk factors supportive of involvement of a soil-borne agent[26,27]	
• Inverse association between disease risk and systemic concentration of antibodies against *C botulinum* bacteria and toxin[28]	• Neuropathology apparently inconsistent with action of *C botulinum* neurotoxins[32]
• Higher mucosal IgA against BoNT/C and D in patients with acute ED vs control animals[29]	• SNARE protein expression in ED ganglion and enteric neurons inconsistent with action of *C botulinum* neurotoxins[32]
	• Lack of evidence of temporal and geographic clustering of ED and neuroparalytic botulism cases

Abbreviation: IgA, immunoglobulin A.

Table 2
Factors associated with increased or decreased risk of equine dysautonomia occurring or recurring on the same premise or that are associated with equine dysautonomia

Level	Factor	Increased (↑) or Decreased (↓) Risk
Horse level	Age (2–7 y)[33,34]	↑ (Occ)
	Low serum antibodies to *C botulinum* type C and BoNT/C[28]	↑ (Occ)
	Good body condition[34]	↑ (Occ)
	Contact with a previous patient with ED[33]	↓ (Occ)
Premises level	Previous ED occurrence on premises[26,33]	↑ (Occ)
	High soil nitrogen content[26,37]	↑ (Occ)
	Pasture/soil disturbance[26]	↑ (Occ)
	High number of horses[34]	↑ (Occ)
	Presence of younger animals[27]	↑ (Occ/Rec)
	Stud farms/livery and riding establishments[27]	↑ (Rec)
	Loam and sandy soils[27]	↑ (Rec)
	Rearing of domestic birds[27]	↑ (Rec)
	High herbage iron, lead, arsenic, and chromium[37]	Association
	Abundance of *Ranunculus* spp (buttercups)[37]	Association
	High soil titanium[38]	↑ (Occ)
	Low soil zinc and chromium[38]	↑ (Occ)
	Chalk soil[27]	↓ (Rec)
Management level	Grazing[33,34]	↑ (Occ)
	Recent movement (especially within preceding 2 wk)[33,34]	↑ (Occ)
	Change in feed type/quantity within preceding 2 wk[28]	↑ (Occ)
	Ultimate and penultimate use of an ivermectin-based anthelmintic[28]	↑ (Occ)
	Mechanical removal of feces from pasture[27]	↑ (Rec)
	Manual removal of feces from pasture[27]	↓ (Rec)
	Grass cutting[27]	↓ (Rec)
	Cograzing with ruminants[27]	↓ (Rec)
	Feeding of supplementary hay/haylage[28]	↓ (Occ)
Climate level	Recent (within 10–14 d) cool, dry weather and irregular ground frosts[36]	↑ (Occ)
	Increased sun hours and frost days[36,39]	↑ (Occ)
	Higher average maximum temperature[39]	↓ (Occ)

Abbreviations: Occ, occurring; Rec, recurring.

retrospective consideration will often reveal patients with a more protracted, yet recent change in demeanor, reduction in feed intake, and/or weight loss.

PHYSICAL EXAMINATION

The clinical phenotype of the case is largely determined by the severity of neuronal loss,[40] partly within the ANS but predominantly within the ENS. Consequently, the clinical presentation of severely affected patients will differ quite markedly from that of mildly affected patients, despite an identical neuroanatomical distribution of lesions. Similarly, physical examination findings and ancillary diagnostic test results derived from ED cases of differing severities can often reveal quite disparate results. Consequently, the terms *acute*, *subacute*, and *chronic* are generally applied to reflect severely, moderately, and mildly affected patients, respectively, although one should remain aware that these are relatively arbitrary terms applied to a continuum of disease severities, with inevitable overlap between each. However, adoption of this terminology can be clinically beneficial from a prognostic viewpoint. Because a proportion of patients with chronic ED may survive, their differentiation from acute and subacute cases, which are invariably fatal, is important. **Table 3**, which summarizes the clinical signs associated with the acute/subacute (combined) and chronic ED subcategories, highlights the fact that, although certain clinical findings are common to all 3 subcategories, others are more typical of a specific subcategory. The reader is referred to other publications that cover the clinicopathologic correlates associated with each individual clinical sign in more detail.[23,41,42]

ANCILLARY DIAGNOSTIC TESTS

A variety of ancillary diagnostic tests can significantly improve the diagnostic accuracy when presented with a suspected case of ED. These tests can be considered as (1) reflecting nonspecific hematologic, biochemical, bacteriologic, and/or physiologic consequences of the disease; (2) reflecting the degree of ANS and/or ENS dysfunction; (3) reflecting other neurologic deficits not attributable to ANS/ENS involvement; and (4) providing histopathologic evidence of neuronal degeneration. These tests are summarized in **Table 4**.

Ancillary diagnostic tests can also be applied to specifically exclude other differential diagnoses. With regard to chronic ED, such tests may focus on the elimination of other diseases that present with rapid weight loss. With regard to acute ED cases, which present with small intestinal ileus and gastric reflux, the principal aim is to rule out other conditions with a similar presentation, namely, strangulating and nonstrangulating small intestinal obstructive lesions. Therefore, when presented with acute ED cases, there is a greater degree of investigative urgency to enable the identification of other conditions that may require immediate surgical intervention. Consequently, exploratory laparotomy may be indicated in some acute ED cases, the findings of which will determine the need for further diagnostic approaches.

Given that acute ED carries a hopeless prognosis for survival, the clinician must decide whether the absence of a surgically correctable lesion at laparotomy is sufficient grounds for euthanasia by ruling out physical obstructions of the small intestine and failing to provide any beneficial surgical intervention. Alternatively, more confirmatory diagnostic evidence may be warranted before making this decision. Although histopathologic examination of an appropriately sized formalin-fixed ileal biopsy is 100% diagnostically sensitive and specific,[54] this requires a sufficient period of time for tissue fixing, thus, necessitating recovery from anesthesia pending results of the examination. Unfortunately, histopathologic examination of cryostat sections is not 100% specific (because of processing artifacts), thus, risking an erroneous diagnosis and potentially an inappropriate euthanasia.[54]

POSTMORTEM DIAGNOSTIC CONFIRMATION

Postmortem diagnostic confirmation is warranted given the potential risk to other grazing horses on the premises. Implementing short- and long-term risk-avoidance strategies (see later) can be expensive and labor intensive and understandably more justifiable when ED is confirmed. Gross pathologic findings generally reflect the extent of involvement of the ENS. For example, fluid distension of the small intestine and stomach and linear ulceration of the distal esophagus are typical findings in acute ED, whereas patients with subacute ED will have firm corrugated impactions of the large colon and cecum, typically with a black coating on the surface of the firm ingesta.[23,41] Patients with chronic ED are typically emaciated with scant intestinal

Table 3
Clinical signs associated with the 3 subcategories of equine dysautonomia (acute and subacute equine dysautonomia [combined] and chronic equine dysautonomia)

Clinical Sign	Acute/Subacute ED	Chronic ED
Dull demeanor	Present: generally more prevalent sign than moderate/severe colic	Present: generally less severe than acute/subacute ED
Reduced appetite	Acute: usually profoundly anorexic Subacute: variable	Common but variable severity and often progressive in the early stages of disease
Clinical dehydration	Often apparent in acute ED, less so in subacute ED	Mild in some cases, depending on degree of dysphagia
Tachycardia	Acute: typically 80–120 bpm Subacute: typically 60–80 bpm	Typically 45–60 bpm
Bilateral ptosis	Almost invariably present	Almost invariably present
Hypersalivation	Acute: often marked intermittent drooling evident, no nasal return of saliva or food Subacute: rarely present	Not a feature of chronic ED
Dysphagia	Often profoundly dysphagic, although can be difficult to recognize if anorexic	Varying degrees of dysphagia; valuable prognostic indicator
Rhinitis sicca	Acute: rarely appreciable Subacute: may detect slight drying and hyperemia of the nasal mucosa	Variable severity Over time, large casts develop within nasal cavities resulting in stertor Inverse relationship with appetite
Sweating	Varies from patchy to generalized	Patchy sweating May worsen during periods of excitement/anxiety
Abdominal pain	Inconsistently present; if present, usually mild to moderate Not consistent with degree of tachycardia	Usually absent; if present, usually intermittent (eg, postprandial) and mild
Intestinal sounds	Often complete absence of intestinal sounds	Usually reduced, rarely absent
Abdominal shape	Occasional abdominal distension due to large intestinal tympany	Rapid development of characteristic tucked-up abdominal silhouette (greyhoundlike appearance)
Muscle tremors	Muscle tremors over triceps, flanks, and quadriceps	Muscle tremors over triceps, flanks, and quadriceps
Rectal temperature	Normal or elevated rectal temperature (up to 40°C)	Normal or mild elevation in rectal temperature
Stance	Acute: normal stance Subacute: may develop base-narrow stance over a few days	Base-narrow (elephant on a tub) stance
Other clinical signs		Paraphimosis in entire males (less common in geldings) Esophageal choke and aspiration pneumonia may develop as secondary complication of dysphagia

Abbreviation: bpm, beats per minute.

Table 4
Ancillary diagnostic tests that can be used in the diagnostic approach to suspected cases of equine dysautonomia

Diagnostic Test Objective	Diagnostic Test	Comment
Identification of nonspecific ED-associated hematologic, biochemical, physiologic, and/or bacteriologic abnormalities	Increased hematocrit[43]	Reflective of total body water loss (eg, small intestinal sequestration [acute ED], neurogenic impairment of drinking)
	Elevated serum urea concentration[43]	Reflective of total body water loss
	Elevated serum acute phase protein concentration[44,45]	Reflective of systemic inflammatory response
	Elevated urine specific gravity, protein, and creatinine concentration[46]	Reflective of attempted water retention (see previous)
	Elevated peritoneal fluid specific gravity and protein concentration[47,48]	
	Fecal C perfringens detection (ELISA)[30]	Considered to reflect nonspecific clostridial overgrowth in dysmotile bowel
Identification of ANS and/or ENS dysfunction	Temporary reversal of ptosis following topical application of 0.5% phenylephrine ophthalmic solution to the conjunctival sac[49,50]	Confirms neurogenic smooth muscle paralysis (Müller superior tarsal muscle) as the mechanism underlying the ptosis
	Barium swallow study[51]	Retrograde flow reflecting abnormal/uncoordinated esophageal motility
	Esophagoscopy[41]	Evidence of retrograde flow of gastric fluid, either visualized or reflected by the presence of distal esophageal linear ulceration
	Nasogastric intubation[41]	Voluminous foul smelling gastric fluid reflux, potentially reflective of severe gastrointestinal ileus (acute ED)
	Abdominal ultrasonography[41]	Distended small intestinal loops visible, potentially reflective of generalized gastrointestinal ileus (acute ED)
	Transrectal palpation[41]	Distended small intestinal loops palpable, potentially reflective of generalized gastrointestinal ileus (acute ED)
		Firm corrugated colonic and cecal contents, potentially reflective of large intestinal ileus and desiccation of fibrous ingesta
Identification of non-ANS/ENS neurologic dysfunction	Electromyography[52]	Reported findings considered consistent with skeletal muscle neuropathy

(continued on next page)

Table 4
(continued)

Diagnostic Test Objective	Diagnostic Test	Comment
Histopathologic evidence of neuropathology at appropriate anatomic sites	Histopathology of ileal biopsy (standard H&E staining)[53]	Evidence of neuronal loss and chromatolysis within myenteric and submucous plexuses Formalin fixed: 100% sensitive and specific[54] Cryostat sections: suboptimal (73%) specificity (false positives resulting from processing artifacts)[54]
	Histopathology of ileal biopsy (synaptophysin immunostaining)[55]	Combined assessment of neuronal density and intensity of synaptophysin immunostaining: reported 100% sensitivity and specificity
	Histopathology of rectal biopsy (standard H&E staining)[56]	Poor sensitivity (21%) when applied to partial thickness biopsies due to low neuronal density[57]
	Histopathology of rectal biopsy (BAPP immunostaining)[58]	Retrospective application of this approach: 100% sensitivity and specificity Requires prospective validation
	Histopathology of gustatory papillae[59]	Retrospective application of this approach: 100% sensitivity and high specificity (98%) Requires prospective validation

Abbreviations: BAPP, β-amyloid precursor protein; ELISA, enzyme-linked immunosorbent assay; H&E, hematoxylin-eosin.

contents, depending on the appetite and degree of dysphagia at the time of death.[23,41] Bilateral *rhinitis sicca* is commonly seen in chronic ED.

A definitive diagnosis is achieved by histopathologic examination of autonomic (prevertebral and paravertebral) ganglia and intestinal ENS plexuses (see earlier discussion).[60,61] Autonomic ganglia most routinely collected for histopathologic examination include the cranial cervical ganglia, the cranial and caudal mesenteric ganglia, and the abdominal and thoracic sympathetic chain.

Typical histologic features include chromatolysis with loss of Nissl substance, eccentricity or pyknosis of the nuclei, neuronal swelling and vacuolation, accumulation of intracytoplasmic eosinophilic spheroids, and axonal dystrophy.[60–63]

TREATMENT OF CHRONIC EQUINE DYSAUTONOMIA: SELECTION OF CANDIDATES

As previously stated, most ED cases have a hopeless prognosis. Overall, ED is associated with an approximately 80% mortality: comprising 100% mortality in acute and subacute ED and approximately 50% mortality in chronic ED.[64,65] Therefore, the selection of candidates for treatment relies firstly on subcategorizing the case (see **Table 2**) and, secondly, if the signs are consistent with chronic ED, selecting the appropriate patients for which treatment is indicated. Acute and subacute ED cases are invariably fatal[23]; however, supportive care (not covered in this review) in the form of intravenous (IV) fluid infusion, analgesic administration, and regular gastric decompression may be initiated to stabilize patients until a more definitive diagnosis is achieved, at which point euthanasia is indicated.

The criteria used for the selection of appropriate patients with chronic ED are relatively arbitrary; however, the following list is a useful guide:

- Ability to swallow, albeit compromised
- Some remaining appetite, albeit markedly reduced
- Absence of continuous moderate to severe abdominal pain (rarely will patients with chronic ED exhibit severe colic)

Additionally, in light of the prolonged period of convalescence required in many cases,[64,65] an appropriate level of commitment should be declared by the owners: either time commitment if they opt for home nursing or financial commitment if they opt to refer to a clinical facility for nursing care.

NONPHARMACOLOGIC TREATMENT OPTIONS FOR CHRONIC EQUINE DYSAUTONOMIA

Treatment of chronic ED is predominantly intensive nursing care. Assuming the aforementioned selection criteria are met, the greatest obstacle to survival is typically profound inappetance.[23] Consequently, the main aim of the nursing care is to attain an adequate level of voluntary feed intake. This target generally involves the provision of a selection of highly palatable feeds (ideally high in energy and protein). As individual preferences change regularly, it is often necessary to offer a variety of feed components and consistencies.[41,66] Although the addition of succulents (eg, carrots, apples) to the diet may improve voluntary feed intake, these alone are insufficient to meet the animal's energy and protein requirements. Feeding small amounts regularly reduces waste and is more likely to result in a greater overall feed intake over a 24-hour period. At the authors' institute, newly hospitalized patients with chronic ED receive 2 hourly small feeds, reducing to 4 hourly feeds after approximately 1 week of hospitalization. Both continuous-flow enteral feeding and total and partial parenteral nutrition have been used in selected patients, with little evidence of a positive influence on patient outcomes.[67] However, via a reduction in the initial rate of weight loss, their use may extend the period of time available for a spontaneous improvement in appetite to occur. Additional nonpharmacologic approaches include regular hand grazing and light exercise in the form of in-hand walking and/or short periods of turn out to pasture.

PHARMACOLOGIC TREATMENT OPTIONS FOR CHRONIC EQUINE DYSAUTONOMIA

Pharmacologic treatment options in chronic ED can be subcategorized as follows:

Appetite Stimulants

Unfortunately, attempts to pharmacologically improve the appetite of patients with chronic ED have been unrewarding, as determined by both anecdotal evidence and placebo-controlled trials.[68] Evaluated drugs include glucocorticoids, brotizalam, diazepam, and cyproheptadine.

Prokinetics

Administration of the prokinetic drug cisapride has been shown to increase dry matter intake and decrease gastrointestinal transit time.[69] However, as the principal reason for treatment failure is a lack of voluntary feed intake and not intestinal dysmotility, the use of such motility-enhancing drugs is rarely indicated. Furthermore, by definition, patients with chronic ED have sufficiently coordinated intestinal motility to maintain an aboral flow of ingesta.

Analgesics

The judicious use of nonsteroidal antiinflammatory drugs (NSAIDs) is often beneficial. The analgesic properties of these drugs can be useful to combat low-grade, intermittent (often postprandial) abdominal pain. Furthermore, as patients with ED have evidence of low-grade systemic inflammation (eg, elevated acute phase proteins),[44,45] the antiinflammatory properties of this class of drugs are theoretically beneficial. Appropriate NSAID therapeutic options include flunixin meglumine (0.5 mg/kg by mouth or IV twice a day) or phenylbutazone (2.2 mg/kg by mouth or IV twice a day).

Antimicrobials

The dysphagia present in most patients with chronic ED may result in varying degrees of aspiration. In such cases, broad-spectrum antimicrobial administration is indicated to minimize the development of inhalation pneumonia. Commonly adopted empirical antimicrobial treatments include oxytetracycline (10 mg/kg IV once a day), combined gentamicin (6.6 mg/kg IV once a day) and procaine penicillin (12 mg/kg intramuscularly twice a day), and trimethoprim sulfonamide (15–30 mg/kg by mouth twice a day). Occasionally, metronidazole (20 mg/kg by mouth 3 times a day) may also be indicated when anaerobic infection is suspected.

TREATMENT COMPLICATIONS AND PROGNOSTIC INDICATORS

Although it can be difficult to predict the response to treatment/nursing early in the disease process, several factors can be used as potential prognostic indicators. These factors are itemized next:

Appetite

Although the voluntary feed intake of patients can fluctuate markedly over a 24-hour or 48-hour period, persistence of complete anorexia for several (eg, 5) consecutive days is generally a poor prognostic indicator, provided that several feed options have been offered. Persistent anorexia and associated weight loss and weakness remain the principal reasons for euthanasia in patients receiving nursing care.

Magnitude and Rate of Weight Loss

A recent retrospective study of hospitalized patients with chronic ED demonstrated the prognostic value of considering the magnitude and rate of weight loss over specific periods of treatment. Survival prediction curves have the potential to offer useful prospective prognostic information on individual patients.[65]

Rhinitis Sicca

Studies have identified an inverse association between survival and the severity of rhinitis sicca.[70] It is hypothesized that severe rhinitis sicca will directly and negatively influence appetite, potentially via an effect on olfaction.

Inhalation Pneumonia

Some patients with chronic ED with severe dysphagia may develop inhalation pneumonia as a consequence of aspiration of food, saliva and rhinitis sicca casts. It is worth noting that coughing seems to be a poor indicator of this complication; rather, patients become pyrexic and increasingly dull and with inappetence. Consequently, recognition of this complication often depends on regular ultrasonographic examinations of the cranioventral thorax, assessing for the presence of lung consolidation and occasionally pleural fluid accumulation.

Fulminant Diarrhea

Severe diarrhea has been recognized in a proportion of patients with chronic ED, usually those receiving supplementary liquid enteral feeding via a nasogastric tube.[67] Fulminant diarrhea is a recognized complication of enteral feeding in horses, thought to partly reflect the low fiber content of commercially available liquid feeds.[71] However, this complication has also been recorded in patients receiving alfalfa slurries, whereby a bacterial overgrowth in the cecum and large colon was suspected. Consequently, when adopted in the treatment of patients with ED, enteral feeding should be introduced gradually and the liquid feed should contain as high a fiber content as feasible.

LONG-TERM COMPLICATIONS

Clinical recovery is generally assumed if patients regain an appetite and body weight. Although most recovered patients will return to their previous level of performance, some residual problems have been reported. These problems include poor exercise tolerance, persistent low-grade dysphagia, recurrent esophageal obstruction, occasional mild colic episodes, and coat changes (piloerection at the site of previous sweating).[64,66,72] Considering that even clinically recovered patients have evidence of extensive neuronal loss in the ENS, it has been hypothesized that clinical recovery may partly be associated with compensatory mechanisms that have restored and maintained an adequate degree of intestinal motility.[73] Interstitial cells of Cajal have been proposed as compensatory cellular candidates.

SUMMARY

ED is a multisystem neuropathy of equids characterized by damage to autonomic, enteric, and somatic neurons. It has an extremely high mortality rate and significant welfare, emotional, and financial consequences. The cause is unknown. Horses with acute or subacute ED, which is invariably fatal, should be euthanized on humane grounds as soon as a confident diagnosis is made. Approximately half of the horses with chronic ED survive with intensive nursing care.

REFERENCES

1. Tocher JF. Grass sickness in horses. Transact Royal Highland Agric Soc 1924;36: 65–83.
2. Schwarz B, Brunthaler R, Hahn C, et al. Outbreaks of equine grass sickness in Hungary. Vet Rec 2012;170:75.
3. Voros K, Bakos Z, Albert M, et al. Occurrence of grass sickness in Hungary. Magy Allatorvosok Lapja 2003;125:67–74.
4. Wlaschitz S, Url A. The first case of chronic grass sickness in Austria. Wien Tierarztl Monatsschr 2004;91:42–5.
5. Eser MW, Feige K, Hilbe M. Clinical signs and diagnosis of acute grass sickness in horses in Switzerland and in Southern Germany. Pferdeheilkunde 2000;16:138–43.
6. Leendertse IP. A horse with grass sickness. Tijdschr Diergeneeskd 1993;118:365–6.
7. Schulze C, Venner M, Pohlenz J. Chronical grass sickness (equine dysautonomia) in a 2 1/2 years old Icelandic mare on a north Frisian island. Pferdeheilkunde 1997;13:345–50.

8. Lhomme C, CollobertLaugier C, Amardeilh MF, et al. Equine dysautonomia: an anatomoclinical study of 8 cases. Rev Med Vet 1996;147:805.
9. Bendixen H. "Grass sickness" in Denmark. Maanedsskr Dyrlaeger 1946;58:41–62.
10. Protopapas KF, Spanoudes KAM, Diakakis NE, et al. Equine grass sickness in Cyprus: a case report. Turk J Vet Anim Sci 2012;36:85–7.
11. Melkova P, Cizek P, Ludvikova E, et al. Equine grass sickness in the Czech Republic: a case report. Vet Med 2014;59:137–40.
12. Woods JA, Gilmour JS. A suspected case of grass sickness in the Falkland Islands. Vet Rec 1991;128:359–60.
13. Stewart WJ. Case of suspected acute grass sickness in a thoroughbred mare. Aust Vet J 1977;53:196.
14. Wright A, Beard L, Bawa B, et al. Dysautonomia in a six-year-old mule in the United States. Equine Vet J 2010;42:170–3.
15. Araya O, Vits L, Paredes E, et al. Grass sickness in horses in southern Chile. Vet Rec 2002;150:695–7.
16. Uzal FA, Doxey DL, Robles CA, et al. Histopathology of the brain stem nuclei of horses with mal seco, an equine dysautonomia. J Comp Pathol 1994;111: 297–301.
17. Uzal FA, Robles CA. Mal seco, a grass sickness-like syndrome of horses in Argentina. Vet Res Commun 1993;17:449–57.
18. Uzal FA, Robles CA, Olaechea FV. Histopathological changes in the coeliaco-mesenteric ganglia of horses with mal seco, a grass sickness-like syndrome, in Argentina. Vet Rec 1992;130:244–6.
19. Cottrell DF, McGorum BC, Pearson GT. The neurology and enterology of equine grass sickness: a review of basic mechanisms. Neurogastroenterol Motil 1999; 11:79–92.
20. Hunter LC, Miller JK, Poxton IR. The association of Clostridium botulinum type C with equine grass sickness: a toxicoinfection? Equine Vet J 1999;31:492–9.
21. Poxton IR, Hunter L, Lough H, et al. Is equine grass sickness (Mal seco?) a form of botulism? Anaerobe 1999;5:291–3.
22. Poxton IR, Hunter LC, Brown R, et al. Clostridia and equine grass sickness. Rev Med Microbiol 1997;8:S49–51.
23. Pirie RS, Jago RC, Hudson NPH. Equine grass sickness. Equine Vet J 2014;46: 545–53.
24. Pirie RS, McGorum BC. Equine grass sickness: benefits of a multifaceted research approach. Equine Vet J 2016;48:770–2.
25. Tocher JF, Tocher JW,F, Brown W. Grass sickness investigation report. Vet Rec 1923;3:37–45.
26. McCarthy HE, French NP, Edwards GB, et al. Why are certain premises at increased risk of equine grass sickness? A matched case-control study. Equine Vet J 2004;36:130–4.
27. Newton JR, Hedderson EJ, Adams VJ, et al. An epidemiological study of risk factors associated with the recurrence of equine grass sickness (dysautonomia) on previously affected premises. Equine Vet J 2004;36:105–12.
28. McCarthy HE, French NP, Edwards GB, et al. Equine grass sickness is associated with low antibody levels to Clostridium botulinum: a matched case-control study. Equine Vet J 2004;36:123–9.
29. Nunn FG, Pirie RS, Mcgorum B, et al. Preliminary study of mucosal IgA in the equine small intestine: specific IgA in cases of acute grass sickness and controls. Equine Vet J 2007;39:457–60.

30. Waggett BE, McGorum BC, Wernery U, et al. Prevalence of Clostridium perfringens in faeces and ileal contents from grass sickness affected horses: comparisons with 3 control populations. Equine Vet J 2010;42:494–9.

31. Garrett LA, Brown R, Poxton IR. A comparative study of the intestinal microbiota of healthy horses and those suffering from equine grass sickness. Vet Microbiol 2002;87:81–8.

32. McGorum BC, Scholes S, Milne EM, et al. Equine grass sickness, but not botulism, causes autonomic and enteric neurodegeneration and increases soluble N-ethylmaleimide-sensitive factor attachment receptor protein expression within neuronal perikarya. Equine Vet J 2016;48:786–91.

33. Wood JLN, Milne EM, Doxey DL. A case-control study of grass sickness (equine dysautonomia) in the United Kingdom. Vet J 1998;156:7–14.

34. Doxey DL, Gilmour JS, Milne EM. A comparative-study of normal equine populations and those with grass sickness (dysautonomia) in eastern Scotland. Equine Vet J 1991;23:365–9.

35. French NP, McCarthy HE, Diggle PJ, et al. Clustering of equine grass sickness cases in the United Kingdom: a study considering the effect of position-dependent reporting on the space-time K-function. Epidemiol Infect 2005;133:343–8.

36. Doxey DL, Gilmour JS, Milne EM. The relationship between meteorological features and equine grass sickness (dysautonomia). Equine Vet J 1991;23:370–3.

37. Edwards SE, Martz KE, Rogge A, et al. Edaphic and phytochemical factors as predictors of equine grass sickness cases in the UK. Front Pharmacol 2010;1:122.

38. Wylie CE, Shaw DJ, Fordyce FM, et al. Equine grass sickness in Scotland: a case-control study of environmental geochemical risk factors. Equine Vet J 2016;48:779–85.

39. Wylie CE, Shaw DJ, Fordyce FM, et al. Equine grass sickness in Scotland: a case-control study of signalment- and meteorology-related risk factors. Equine Vet J 2014;46(1):64–71.

40. Hahn CN, Mayhew IG, de Lahunta A. Central neuropathology of equine grass sickness. Acta Neuropathol 2001;102:153–9.

41. Lyle C, Pirie RS. Equine grass sickness. In Pract 2009;31:26–32.

42. Pirie RS. Grass sickness. Clin Tech Equine Pract 2006;5(1):30–6.

43. Doxey DL, Milne EM, Gilmour JS, et al. Clinical and biochemical features of grass sickness (equine dysautonomia). Equine Vet J 1991;23:360–4.

44. Copas VEN, Durham AE, Stratford CH, et al. In equine grass sickness, serum amyloid A and fibrinogen are elevated, and can aid differential diagnosis from non-inflammatory causes of colic. Vet Rec 2013;172:395.

45. Milne EM, Doxey DL, Kent JE, et al. Acute phase proteins in grass sickness (equine dysautonomia). Res Vet Sci 1991;50:273–8.

46. Fintl C, Milne EM, McGorum BC. Evaluation of urinalysis as an aid in the diagnosis of equine grass sickness. Vet Rec 2002;151:721–4.

47. Milne E. Peritoneal fluid analysis for the differentiation of medical and surgical colic in horses. In Pract 2004;26:444–9.

48. Milne EM, Doxey DL, Gilmour JS. Analysis of peritoneal fluid as a diagnostic aid in grass sickness (equine dysautonomia). Vet Rec 1990;127:162–5.

49. Hahn CN, Mayhew IG. Phenylephrine eye drops as a diagnostic test in equine grass sickness. Vet Rec 2000;147:603–6.

50. Hahn CN, Mayhew IG. Studies on the experimental induction of ptosis in horses. Vet J 2000;160:220–4.

51. Greet TRC, Whitwell KE. Barium swallow as an aid to the diagnosis of grass sickness. Equine Vet J 1986;18:294–7.

52. Wijnberg ID, Franssen H, Jansen GH, et al. The role of quantitative electromyography (EMG) in horses suspected of acute and chronic grass sickness. Equine Vet J 2006;38:230–7.

53. Scholes SFE, Vaillant C, Peacock P, et al. Diagnosis of grass sickness by ileal biopsy. Vet Rec 1993;133:7–10.

54. Milne EM, Pirie RS, McGorum BC, et al. Evaluation of formalin-fixed ileum as the optimum method to diagnose equine dysautonomia (grass sickness) in simulated intestinal biopsies. J Vet Diagn Invest 2010;22:248–52.

55. Waggett BE, McGorum BC, Shaw DJ, et al. Evaluation of synaptophysin as an immunohistochemical marker for equine grass sickness. J Comp Pathol 2010; 142:284–90.

56. Wales AD, Whitwell KE. Potential role of multiple rectal biopsies in the diagnosis of equine grass sickness. Vet Rec 2006;158:372–7.

57. Mair TS, Kelley AM, Pearson GR. Comparison of ileal and rectal biopsies in the diagnosis of equine grass sickness. Vet Rec 2011;168:266.

58. Jago RC, Scholes S, Mair TS, et al. Histological assessment of β-amyloid protein precursor immunolabelled rectal biopsies aids diagnosis of equine grass sickness. Equine Vet J 2018;50:22–8.

59. McGorum BC, Pirie RS, Shaw D, et al. Neuronal chromatolysis in the subgemmal plexus of gustatory papillae in horses with grass sickness. Equine Vet J 2016;48: 773–8.

60. Obel A. Studies on grass disease: the morphological picture with special reference to the vegetative nervous system. J Comp Pathol 1955;65:334–46.

61. Scholes SFE, Vaillant C, Peacock P, et al. Enteric neuropathy in horses with grass sickness. Vet Rec 1993;132:647–51.

62. Brownlee A. Changes in the coeliaco-mesenteric ganglia of horses affected with grass sickness and of horses affected with some other diseases. Vet Rec 1959; 71:668–9.

63. Gilmour JS. Chromatolysis and axonal dystrophy in autonomic nervous system in grass sickness of equidae. Neuropathol Appl Neurobiol 1975;1:39–47.

64. Doxey DL, Milne EM, Harter A. Recovery of horses from dysautonomia (grass sickness). Vet Rec 1995;137:585–8.

65. Jago RC, Handel I, Hahn CN, et al. Bodyweight change aids prediction of survival in chronic equine grass sickness. Equine Vet J 2016;48:792–7.

66. Doxey DL, Tothill S, Milne EM, et al. Patterns of feeding and behavior in horses recovering from dysautonomia (grass sickness). Vet Rec 1995;137:181–3.

67. Pirie RS, Jago RC. Nutritional support for the dysphagic adult horse. Equine Vet Educ 2015;27:430–41.

68. Fintl C, McGorum BC. Evaluation of three ancillary treatments in the management of equine grass sickness. Vet Rec 2002;151:381–3.

69. Milne EM, Doxey DL, Woodman MP, et al. An evaluation of the use of cisapride in horses with chronic grass sickness (equine dysautonomia). Br Vet J 1996;152:537–49.

70. Milne EM, Woodman MP, Doxey DL. Use of clinical measurements to predict the outcome in chronic cases of grass sickness (equine dysautonomia). Vet Rec 1994;134:438–40.

71. Morris DD. Assisted enteral feeding in adult horses. Compendium on Continuing Education for the Practicing Veterinarian 2004;26:46–9.

72. Doxey DL, Milne EM, Ellison J, et al. Long-term prospects for horses with grass sickness (dysautonomia). Vet Rec 1998;142:207–9.

73. Doxey DL, Johnston P, Hahn C, et al. Histology in recovered cases of grass sickness. Vet Rec 2000;146:645–6.

Toxic Causes of Intestinal Disease in Horses

Bryan L. Stegelmeier, DVM, PhD*, T. Zane Davis, PhD

KEYWORDS

- Toxin • Poisoning • Enteritis • Poisonous plant • Toxic plant • Horse • Equine

KEY POINTS

- Most ingested toxins produce enterocyte damage, but these changes are overshadowed by other clinical and organ-specific lesions.
- Arsenic and mercury toxicities are characterized by hemorrhagic enteritis.
- Some plant awns cause oral and mucosal ulceration, irritation, or obstruction.
- Other plant toxins are highly cytotoxic and produce extensive gastroenteritis and colic.
- Some plant toxins produce intestinal fibrosis and colic.

INTRODUCTION

Most toxins are ingested and the gastrointestinal enterocytes are literally the first to be exposed and damaged. However, because many toxins cause extensive organ-specific damage, the gastrointestinal lesions are lost in the shadows of other lesions that have been generally accepted as characteristic of poisoning. A typical example is the microcystin. The microcystins poison horses, cattle, and various other animals including man. They are potent hepatotoxins produced by *Microcystis aeruginosa*, *M viridis*, and *M wesenbergii*. They inhibit cellular serine and threonine protein phosphatases, resulting in excessive phosphorylation of cell regulatory proteins and cytoskeleton collapse. This damage is seen as massive hepatocellular degeneration and necrosis. The disrupted hepatic vascular plate results in hemorrhage and embolization of necrotic and degenerative hepatocytes to distant vessels. Microcystins target hepatocytes as they are absorbed from the portal circulation by bile acid–like receptors. Similar receptors are responsible for microcystin absorption in the ileum where enterocytes have similar receptors. Microcystin's effect in these enterocytes produces extensive degeneration, necrosis, and loss of structure including villous blunting and collapse. However, this damage is rarely identified in poisoned animals because

Disclosure: The authors have no conflict of interest or commercial involvement with this information.

USDA/ARS Poisonous Plant Research Laboratory, 1150 East 1400 North, Logan, UT 84341, USA
* Corresponding author.
E-mail address: bryan.stegelmeier@ars.usda.gov

it is easily misinterpreted as autolytic change or simply overlooked. Similar intestinal lesions are often overlooked in many other poisonings and it is beyond the scope of this article to describe all the toxins that damage the gastrointestinal system or alter its function. The objectives of this article are to review select toxins and poisonous plants that primarily cause gastrointestinal disease in horses.

TOXIN-INDUCED INTESTINAL DISEASE

Heavy metals rarely poison horses and, when they do, they are generally caused by medicinal or diet misformulation (mercury, selenium), contaminated pastures (lead, zinc, arsenic), or contaminated water (cadmium). All heavy metals produce gastro-intestinal lesions with colic and hemorrhagic enteritis; however, most also produce extensive neurologic disease or nephrosis, making the intestinal lesions seem minor in comparison. For example, lead, which is the most common heavy metal that poisons horses, produces severe neurologic disease with prominent laryngeal paralysis. The gastrointestinal lesions are largely overlooked. The exceptions are arsenic and inorganic mercury, which cause severe gastroenteritis with hemorrhagic diarrhea.

Arsenic poisoning is usually caused by contaminated feed, especially contaminated grain. Many poisonings occur when arsenic-containing chemicals are used as wood preservatives or as dressing on seed grains. Other intoxications occur when arsenic-containing insect dips, orchard insecticides, rodenticides, or arsenic-containing medications are inadvertently ingested or when arsenic-containing medicinals are used inappropriately.[1,2] Arsenic-induced gastroenteritis is characterized by severe necrosis, ulceration, and hemorrhage that results in dehydration, electrolyte imbalances, and acidosis. Poisoning is generally identified by associating clinical signs with a kidney arsenic concentration of greater than 10 ppm. Chronic poisoning can be best characterized using hair analysis. Toxicity is produced when arsenical salts react with cellular sulfhydryl groups on proteins and enzymes, disrupting cellular metabolism, including oxidative phosphorylation. Some arsenicals may directly inhibit oxidative phosphorylation by replacing phosphate in those reactions. Arsenical valence is critical to both site and severity of toxicity. Dose and duration determine the clinical syndrome. High doses generally produce neurologic signs with sudden death. Lesser doses produce gastroenteritis with fetid hemorrhagic diarrhea. Disease may become more severe over several days with neurologic signs and death within 5 or 6 days. Lower doses produce chronic disease affecting mostly the skin and hair, and at times producing chronic conjunctivitis with ulcers. Treatment includes removing the source of exposure and decreasing absorption using laxatives, sodium thiosulfate, or dimercaprol.

Mercury poisoning is uncommon today, because its toxicity is well-known and its use has been discontinued in most medicinal, manufacturing, and industrial processes. Rare equine poisonings have been reported to occur when organic mercuric fungicides were used as seed preservatives or inorganic mercury was used in some blistering agents. The mercury salts are corrosive, producing extensive gastrointestinal necrosis and hemorrhage along with renal tubular necrosis. When mercuric salts were used medicinally, oral ulcers were historically used to monitor "effectiveness" of the purported treatment. Clinically, poisoning is characterized by diarrhea with anorexia and nervousness. There are also clinical urinalysis changes of renal failure including glycosuria, proteinuria, phospaturia, isothenuria, polyuria with granular casts, and increased urinary gamma-glutamyl transpeptidase, alkaline phosphatase, and amino aspartate transferase activities. Histologic changes include extensive renal tubular necrosis with necrotizing and hemorrhagic enteritis. When poisoned, the kidney and liver have the highest mercury concentrations, suggesting that these are good samples for diagnostic analysis. In addition to nephrosis and gastroenteritis, mercury poisoning in some horses can produce granulomatous lesions in the lungs, kidneys, liver, and bone marrow. The pathogenesis of these lesions is not understood.[2] Treatment of mercury poisoning includes diuresis with extensive fluid therapy and removal of exposure (such as to blistering agents). It has been suggested that a chelating agent such as N-acetyl-DL-penicillamine can accelerate toxin clearance.

Various medications such as nonsteroidal antiinflammatory drugs and anticholinesterases such as neostigmine, edrophonium, pyridostigmine, or various organophosphates (parathion, malathion, etc) all produce diarrhea and may be associated with focal mucosal ulcerations. As with the heavy metal intoxications, most of these gastrointestinal lesions are largely overlooked in the shadow of prominent neurologic disease.

POISONOUS PLANTS THAT CAUSE GASTROINTESTINAL DISEASE
Mechanical Damage

There are various grasses (foxtails [*Setaria, Alopecurus, Bromus,* and *Hordeum* spp.], needle grasses [*Stipa* spp.], squirrel tail [*Sitanion hystrix*], bristle grass [*Setaria lutescens*], medusa head rye [*Taentherum Asperum*], prairie 3-awn [*Aristida oligantha*], tanglehead [*Heteropogon contortus*], triticale [*Triticosecale* spp.], sandburs [*Cenchrus* spp.], cheatgrasses [*Bromus* spp.; **Fig. 1**] and others) that cause mechanical damage as they injure mucosal surfaces of the mouth, eyes, ears, skin folds, and migrate through soft tissues. These migrations make the plant material difficult to find and remove surgically. These weedy plants often expand and dominate fields, ranges, and pastures when they are overgrazed or not properly managed. When mature, the seeds have spine- covered awns that can irritate, penetrate, and migrate into mucosal surfaces, skin folds, and soft tissues. These grasses are poor-quality forages and usually are not palatable when they are mature; however, horses eat them when there are no alternative forages or when they are included in hay or other prepared feeds. As suggested, the mature grass awns are ingested and become embedded in the mucous membranes of the gums and tongue, causing ulcers and abscesses.

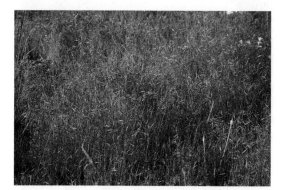

Fig. 1. Cheat grass (*Bromus tectorum*) is an annual invasive grass native to Euroasia that invades and often dominates pastures, fields, and rangelands. Cheat grass germinates in the fall or spring with rapid growth, flowering, and seed production in the spring and early summer. Horses avoid grazing free standing cheat grass if alternative forages are available but, as with many irritating grasses, they will eat them when they are included in hay.

Affected horses salivate excessively and have difficulty eating. The economic impact is large because affected animals are reluctant to eat, lose condition, and extensive care is required to extract the plant material, drain and clean wounds, and maintain appropriate antibiotic therapy.[3] Larger plant awns and burrs also can cause gastrointestinal obstruction and colic. Avoiding contaminated hay and maintaining pastures to avoid exposure is recommended.

Obstruction

Some plants have indigestible fibers, burrs, and some poorly identified plant parts that bind or coagulate with plant material, hair, and debris that harden as they accumulate magnesium ammonium phosphate. The resulting concretions have been termed phytoconglobates or phytobezoars (**Fig. 2**). Such phytobezoars can be single or multiple and they may weigh up to 10 kg. These concretions persist in the gastrointestinal tract, especially in the equine colon, where they increase in size until they intermittently or permanently obstruct colonic function and flow. Although all the plants and physiologic conditions have not been identified completely that contribute to phytobezoar production, several plants have been associated with phytobezoar production. These plants include German millet and Hungarian grass (*Setaria* spp.), Australian onion grass (*Romulea rosea*), Oat chaff (*Arena saliva*), and American persimmon (*Diospyros virginiana*). Of these plants, persimmon has the highest association because it has been reported to cause epidemic outbreaks of equine gastric phytobezoars and colic. In most cases, affected horses present with colic and, although some enteroliths can be detected via rectal palpation, most are not discovered until the stomach or colon is inspected surgically or at necropsy. Consequently, treatment is generally supportive. Persimmon gastric phytobezoars have been successfully treated with cellulose, mineral oil, and even cola soft drinks, along with changing the diet to a pelleted feed to dissolve these concretions.[4] As suggested, other plants that have large seeds, tubers, or burs cause obstruction and choke in ruminants, but these plants rarely cause problems in horses because they are more discriminating and more carefully chew their food.

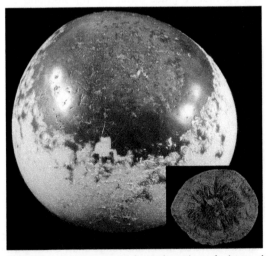

Fig. 2. This 19-cm phytobezoar was removed from the colon of a horse that died from colic. This was the only one found in this horse, but occasionally there may be numerous phytobezoars of varying size.

Stomatitis and Gastroenteritis

There are several different nightshades that are all *Solanum* species. Nightshades that poison livestock include *S rostratum* (buffalo bur), *S ptycanthum* or *nigrum* (black nightshade), *S dulcamara* (bittersweet nightshade; **Fig. 3**), *S elaeagnifolium* (silverleaf nightshade), *S carolinense* (Carolina horse nettle), *S dimidiatum* (western horse nettle), and *S triflorum* (cutleaf nightshade). These plants produce several toxic syndromes because they contain both steroidal glycoalkaloids that cause severe gastroenteritis and cholinesterase inhibitors that produce neurologic disease. In horses, poisoning is similarly mixed. *S triflorum* poisoning in horses produces primarily a stomatitis with extensive hypersalivation (**Fig. 4**).[5] This can be contrasted with *S carolinense*, which produces neurologic disease that can be potentiated by ivermectin therapy.[6] The indicator *Solanum* steroidal glycoalkaloid has been identified as solanine, a potent mucosal irritant that commonly causes stomatitis. Solanine concentrations can be high, especially in berries. Toxic silver leaf nightshade berries are lethal at doses as small as 0.1% to 0.3% of body weight. Clinical poisoning includes anorexia, salivation, abdominal pain, diarrhea, dilation of pupils, dullness, depression, weakness, progressive paralysis, prostration, and rarely death. Treatment generally is symptomatic with use of fluid therapy, activated charcoal, and cautious use of cholinergics such as physostigmine. Some *Solanum* spp. invade into fields and commonly contaminate hay (**Fig. 5**), were they can poison livestock.[5]

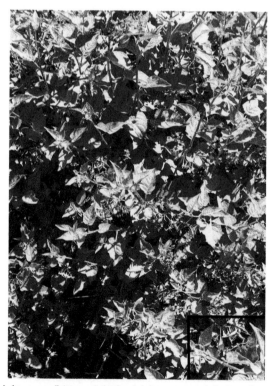

Fig. 3. *Solanum dulcamara* (bitter nightshade) is a perennial vine that grows over other plants or up fences. The flowers are star shaped with 5 purple petals and yellow stamens. The fruit is an oval red berry about 1 cm long that is toxic for livestock and man.

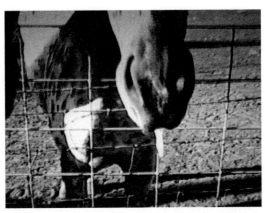

Fig. 4. Horse poisoned with cutleaf nightshade (*Solanum triflora*). This horse was trembling, making photography difficult. Notice the extensive hypersalivation. The mucosal surface (not seen) was red and edematous.

Pokeweed (Phytolacca americana)

Pokeweed (*P americana*) is a perennial branching herb that grows up to 3 m high with green to purple stems, large 20-cm ovate leaves, small white flowers, and shiny green berries that turn purple-black when ripe. Pokeweed is a weedy plant with a deep tap root that provides it drought tolerance. Its weedy nature allows it to infest pastures, expand in marginal areas, and spread along fence lines. All parts of the plant contain saponins, oxalates, and phytolacine, but the roots are the most toxic. The berries may also contain lectins that have immunologic effects. Horses are generally poisoned by eating leaves and stems. When ingested, the response is dose dependent with small doses producing mild stomatitis and hypersalivation with low-grade chronic colic and

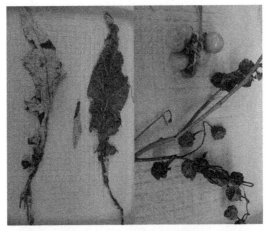

Fig. 5. *Solanum* spp. that was found in hay associated with livestock poisoning. This is most likely Carolina horse nettle (*Solanum carolinense*). Carolina horse nettle is a perennial native of the southeastern United States and now can be found in temperate areas of North America, Europe, Asia, and Australia. The leaves are long and oval, with coarsely toothed edges and fine hairs on both sides. The flowers have 5 white to purple petals with yellow stamen. The fruit are light green with light stripes. As seen in this sample sorted from dried hay, the fruit wrinkles as it dries.

diarrhea. High doses can be fatal but, because *P americana* is less toxic than other *Phytolacca* species, pokeweed-induced mortality tends to be much lower in North America than other countries.[7] Characteristic necropsy lesions include stomatitis and ulcerative gastroenteritis. Pokeweed is not very palatable, so horses with access to good quality forages generally avoid it. Treatment should be supportive.

Ricinus communis (castor bean)

R communis (castor bean; **Fig. 6**) is a Mediterranean plant that was originally used as an ornamental in many temperate climates. In many locations, it has escaped cultivation and become a weed expanding into fields, pastures, and along fence lines, road sides, and marginal lands. Poisoning usually occurs when animals are fed grain or pelleted feeds that are contaminated with castor bean seeds (it is not a true bean). The toxin, ricin, inhibits protein synthesis and it may be antigenic, causing anaphylaxis in sensitive animals. The seeds are highly toxic, especially to horses. As little as 0.1 mg/kg of body weight of well-chewed or ground seeds can be lethal. Most animals develop clinical signs of poisoning 12 to 48 hours after ingestion. Signs include dull appearance, depression, anorexia, thirst, weakness, colic, trembling, sweating, incoordination, difficult breathing, progressive central nervous system depression, fever, bloody diarrhea, convulsions, and death. Treatment is palliative to reduce absorption, including activated charcoal, cathartics, and mineral oil, as well as fluids and steroids as supportive care. Poisoning often is fatal; many animals die without early intervention.[8]

Jimsonweed (Datura stramonium)

Jimsonweed (*D stramonium*; **Fig. 7**) is an American plant that now has worldwide distribution. It has many common names, including Jamestown weed, thornapple, downy thornapple, devil's trumpet, angel's trumpet, mad apple, stink weed, toloache, and tolguacha among others. Jimsonweed is an annual plant that grows up 1.5 m tall. It quickly spreads in disturbed soils and it easily expands into fields, pastures, and marginal lands. It has white or purple trumpetlike flowers and prickly seed capsules. All parts of the jimsonweed plant are poisonous, but the seeds are especially rich in tropane alkaloids. Major alkaloids include hyoscine, L-hyoscine (scopolamine), and hyoscyamine (atropine). Because these substances act as competitive

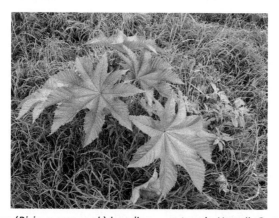

Fig. 6. Castor bean (*Ricinus communis*) invading a pasture in Hawaii. Castor bean is a fast-growing perennial shrub that can grow to 10 m tall. The long leaves (up to 40 cm) are alternate, palmate with 5 to 12 deep lobes with coarsely toothed edges. Young leaves may be reddish and they become dark green as they mature.

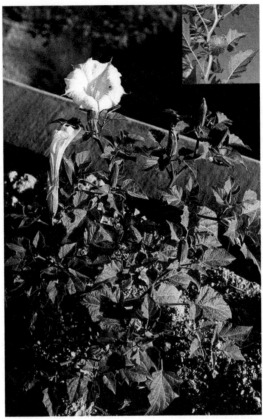

Fig. 7. Jimsonweed *(Datura stramonium)* is an annual from the *Solanaceae* that contains toxic tropane alkaloids. Poisoning generally occurs when animals eat seeds that contaminate grain or dried plant that is harvested with hay. The inset contains immature green Jimsonweed burrs that are 0.5 to 1.5 cm in diameter. These harden and become brown when mature and each contains hundreds of small 0.5- to 1.0-mm black seeds.

antagonists of acetylcholine at peripheral and central muscarinic receptors, poisoning results in the inhibition of parasympathetic innervated tissues. Symptoms of poisoning in horses include a weak and rapid pulse, behavioral changes, dilated pupils, dry mouth, incoordination, diarrhea, colic, convulsions, coma, and sometimes death. It has been suggested that lower doses predispose horses to colic and intestinal impaction.[9,10] Jimsonweed has a foul odor and taste, and horses rarely consume it if they have other forage. However, when it invades fields, it can be harvested with grains. Such contaminated grains and their screenings are highly toxic and should never be fed. Dried plant harvested with hay also remains toxic and has been linked to livestock poisoning.[11] Treatment includes symptomatic therapy and activated charcoal to prevent further absorption. Severely affected animals may benefit from treatment with physostigmine.

Convolvulus arvensis (field bindweed, morning glory)
C arvensis (field bindweed, morning glory; **Fig. 8**) is an extremely persistent, invasive, noxious weed that invades pastures and paddocks. It is a climbing or creeping perennial that grows from 0.5 to 2 m high. It has 2-4 cm, arrowhead-shaped leaves

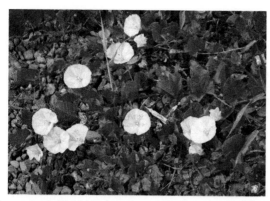

Fig. 8. *Convolvulus arvensis* (field bindweed, morning glory) is a noxious invasive perennial weed. It is prostrate with alternate leaves and pinkish white, funnel-shaped flowers. It spreads using seeds and extensive rhizome systems, making it difficult to control.

and trumpet-shaped white or pink flowers. It produces light brown 0.3-cm fruits that contain 2 seeds. The seeds are robust and remain viable in the soil for 20 years or longer. It proliferates using both seeds and rhizomes and dominates plant communities owing to its rapid, creeping, and choking growth. It often produces dense mats that replace cultivated plants and obstruct agricultural machinery. Similarly, it can dominate pastures, especially over grazed pastures where it displaces nutritious forages. Bindweed-contaminated hay is also toxic. Poisoned horses develop colic characterized by intestinal stasis and flatulence. They may also have tachycardia and dilated pupils. Bindweed-induced changes include diarrhea, colic, gastrointestinal ulceration, and intestinal thickening and fibrosis. The resinoid convolvulin and several tropane alkaloids have been proposed as potential toxins; however, there is little known concerning the required dose or duration of exposure that will produce toxicity.[12] Because poisoning seems to be irreversible, care should be taken to control exposure by controlling bindweed spread and avoiding contaminated hay. Poisoned horses should be removed from the source and treated symptomatically for colic.

Black and New Mexican black locust (Robinia pseudoacacia and R neomexicana)

Black and New Mexican Black Locust (*R pseudoacacia* and *R neomexicana*) are small deciduous trees that grow to just over 20 m. They are North American natives that have been planted and naturalized in Europe, Africa, and Asia. The leaves are compound with paired leaflets on either side of a stem or rachis and a single leaflet at the tip. It has cream-white, pea-like flowers that form showy drooping clumps or racemes that are 10 to 20 cm long. The fruit is a straight, flat, legume-like pod that contains many seeds. Young trees may have thorns that are often not present on the mature trunk or branches. The toxin has been identified as robin, a lectin that is similar to ricin. Horses are poisoned when they eat the seeds or bark, but there are also reports of toxicity relating to bedding animals with black locust sawdust.[13,14] Signs of poisoning include colic, constipation, bloody diarrhea, muscle weakness, laminitis, and irregular heartbeat. In severe cases of black locust poisoning, the horse may have dilated pupils and develop heart irregularities that may be fatal.[15] However, most animals recover with removal of exposure and supportive treatment.

Ranunculus spp

The *Ranunculaceae* family includes the buttercups, which is a rather diverse group of plants that includes both annual and perennial opportunistic plants that expand in disturbed soils like those commonly found in overgrazed horse pastures. In North America, *Ceratocephalus testiculatus* or bur buttercup is the species most often associated with livestock poisoning. Bur buttercup poisoning is most common in sheep; horses generally find it undesirable. Poisoning is characterized by oral irritation seen as blistered lips and stomatitis resulting in increased salivation. More extensive intoxication produces gastroenteritis with colic and diarrhea. Buttercup contains the toxin ranunculin that is converted to protoanemonin, a mucosal irritant.[16] Fresh leaves and flowers are toxic, but they lose toxicity when dried for hay. In severe cases, poisoning

Table 1	
Partial list of toxic plants that contain toxic cardiac glycosides or grayanotoxins	
Cardiac Glycosides	
Acokanthera spp.	Bushman's poison bush
Adenium multiflorum	Impala lily
Adonis microcarpa	Pheasant's eye
Asclepias spp.	Milkweeds
Asclepias curassavica	Red-head cotton bush
Apocynum cannabinum	Dogbane
Bryophyllum spp.	Kalanhoe
Cheiranthus cheiri	Wallflower
Convallaria majalis	Lily of the valley
Corchorus olitorius	Jute
Cryptostegia grandiflora	Rubber vine
Digitalis purpurea and *D lanata*	Foxglove
Euonymus spp.	Euonymus
Gomphocarpus spp.	Milkweed, balloon cotton
Helleborus spp.	Hellebores
Homeria flaccida and *H miniata*	One- and 2-leaf cape tulip
Hyacinthium spp.	Hyacinth
Kalanchoe delagoensis	Mother of millions
Nerium oleander	Oleander
Ornithogalum spp.	Star of Bethlehem
Sisyrinchium spp.	Blue eyed grass
Strophanthus spp.	Poison rope
Thevetia peruviana	Yellow oleander
Urginea spp.	Squill
Vinca major	Periwinkle
Virginea maritima	Squill
Grayanotoxins	
Kalmia latifolia	Mountain laurel
Leucothoe spp.	Fetter bush, black laurel
Lyonia ligustrina	Maleberry
Pieris japonica	Japanese Pieris
Rhododendron spp.	Rhododendron

may lead to convulsions and death. As long as horses have access to adequate pasture or hay, it is unlikely that they will ingest a toxic dose. The other *Ranunculus* spp. that occasionally poison horses in other countries produce a different syndrome that is characterized by prominent neurologic disease.[17,18]

Cardioglycosides (cardenolides and bufadienolides) and grayanotoxins

Although these toxins are very different and have different mechanisms of action, we have grouped them together. Poisonined horses often present with colic and gastroenteritis even though the lethal clinical and pathologic lesions are myotoxic often with cardiac arrhythmias. A select list of these toxic plants is included in **Table 1**. Cardiac glycosides inhibit the membrane sodium–potassium pump in excitable membranes. This inhibition increases the intracellular sodium, which correlates with a change in cardiac contraction by increasing intracellular calcium that can be sequestered in the sarcoplasmic reticulum to be released with subsequent stimulation increasing contraction. Toxic doses result in sodium and potassium imbalances, altered membrane potentials, and if severe atrioventricular block and ventricular fibrillation. Similarly, grayanotoxins bind to sodium channels in cell membrane and prevent inactivation of these sodium channels, similarly resulting in increased intracellular sodium that can produce similar depolarization and myocardial dysfunction. At doses commonly seen in clinical cases, most horses present with colic; however, published reports suggest that grayanotoxin poisoning in horses is less severe and the colic and gastroenteritis are usually much less fatal than with plants containing cardioglycosides. The clinical effect of poisoning in both cases depends on dose and duration. Fatal cardiac glycoside doses cause severe myocardial electrolyte changes that

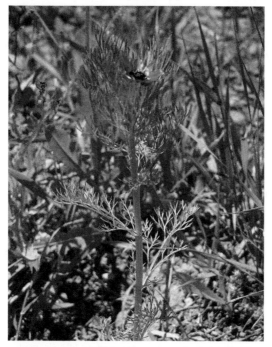

Fig. 9. Pheasant's eye (*Adonis aestivalis*) is a European plant that has become naturalized in many areas, including North America. It is an upright annual that grows from 0.2 to 0.3 m tall. It has orange flowers with fine, carrot-like leaves.

may be difficult to detect and animals quickly die before the myofibers and entire myocardium have time to develop degenerative and inflammatory histologic changes. Horses that ingest lower doses may survive and, although they have significant myocardial dysfunction, the clinical signs primarily are those of colic, diarrhea, and gastroenteritis. For example, horses eating grass hay contaminated with pheasant's eye (*Adonis aestivalis*; **Fig. 9**) presented with signs of colic with gaseous distension and ileus. They all became moribund and either died or were humanely killed. All had subtle myocardial necrosis and neutrophilic myocarditis that surely was the cause of death, but the predominant clinical finding was gaseous colic. Experimental studies in rodents similarly demonstrated gastrointestinal necrosis and hemorrhage as an early dose-related change.[19,20] Certainly these toxins should be considered when animals develop colic and gastroenteritis and exposure to these toxic plants is a possibility.

REFERENCES

1. Pace LW, Turnquist SE, Casteel SW, et al. Acute arsenic toxicosis in five horses. Vet Pathol 1997;34:160–4.

2. Casteel SW. Metal toxicosis in horses. Vet Clin North Am Equine Pract 2001;17: 517–27.

3. Johnson P, LaCarrubba A, Messer N, et al. Ulcerative glossitis and gingivitis associated with foxtail grass awn irritation in two horses. Equine Vet Educ 2012;24:182–6.

4. Banse HE, Gilliam LL, House AM, et al. Gastric and enteric phytobezoars caused by ingestion of persimmon in equids. J Am Vet Med Assoc 2011;239:1110–6.

5. Stegelmeier BL, Lee ST, James LF, et al. Cutleaf nightshade (Solanum trifolorum Nutt.) toxicity in horses and hamsters. In: Panter KE, Wierenga TL, Pfister JA, editors. Poisonous plants: global research and solutions. Wallingford (United Kingdom): CABI; 2007. p. 296–300.

6. Norman TE, Chaffin MK, Norton PL, et al. Concurrent ivermectin and Solanum spp. toxicosis in a herd of horses. J Vet Intern Med 2012;26:1439–42.

7. Valle E, Vergnano D, Nebbia C. Suspected pokeweed (*Phytolacca americana*) poisoning as the cause of progressive cachexia in a Shetland pony. J Equine Vet Sci 2016;42:82–7.

8. Akande TO, Odunsi AA, Akinfala EO. A review of nutritional and toxicological implications of castor bean (Ricinus communis L.) meal in animal feeding systems. J Anim Physiol Anim Nutr (Berl) 2016;100:201–10.

9. Binev R, Valchev I, Nikolov J. Clinical and pathological studies on intoxication in horses from freshly cut Jimson weed (Datura stramonium)-contaminated maize intended for ensiling. J S Afr Vet Assoc 2006;77:215–9.

10. Soler-Rodriguez F, Martin A, Garcia-Cambero JP, et al. Datura stramonium poisoning in horses: a risk factor for colic. Vet Rec 2006;158:132–3.

11. Naude TW, Gerber R, Smith RJ, et al. Datura contamination of hay as the suspected cause of an extensive outbreak of impaction colic in horses. J S Afr Vet Assoc 2005;76:107–12.

12. Todd FG, Stermitz FR, Schultheis P, et al. Tropane alkaloids and toxicity of Convolvulus arvensis. Phytochemistry 1995;39:301–3.

13. Zeitelhack M. Poisoning of horses from sawdust litter in a stable. Prakt Tierarzt 1994;75:437–8.

14. Thursby-Pelham RH. False acacia poisoning in horses. Vet Rec 1999;145:148.

15. Keller H, Dewitz W. Poisoning of 9 horses by the bark of the locust tree (Robinia pseudoacacia). Dtsch Tierarztl Wochenschr 1969;76:115–7 [in German].
16. Olsen JD, Anderson TE, Murphy JC, et al. Bur buttercup poisoning of sheep. J Am Vet Med Assoc 1983;183:538–43.
17. Riekarz J. Buttercup poisoning in a horse. Med Weter 1981;37:658.
18. Griess D, Rech J. Diagnosis of acute poisoning by Ranunculi (*Ranunculus acris* L and *Ficaria ranunculoides* L) in horses. Rev Med Vet (Toulouse) 1997;148:55–9.
19. Stegelmeier BL, Hall JO, Lee ST, et al. Pheasant's eye (Adonis aestavalis) toxicity in livestock and rodents. In: Panter KE, Wierenga TL, Pfister JA, editors. Poisonous plants: global research and solutions. Wallingford (United Kingdom): CABI; 2007. p. 463–7.
20. Woods LW, Filigenzi MS, Booth MC, et al. Summer pheasant's eye (Adonis aestivalis) poisoning in three horses. Vet Pathol 2004;41:215–20.

New Perspectives in Equine Intestinal Parasitic Disease
Insights in Monitoring Helminth Infections

Kurt Pfister, DVM, Dip EVPC[a,b,]*, Deborah van Doorn, DVM, PhD[c]

KEYWORDS

- Equine • Strongyles • *Parascaris* • SAT • TST • Egg counts
- Anthelmintic resistance • Epidemiology

KEY POINTS

- Regular anthelmintic treatment schedules have significantly contributed to the spread of anthelmintic resistance in horse helminths, particularly in small strongyles and *Parascaris*.
- This mass (or strategic) anthelmintic treatment—in most cases without prior diagnosis—was originally developed owing to a lack of larvicidal drugs against *Strongylus vulgaris*.
- This high prevalence of AR and shortening of strongyle egg reappearance period after avermectins/moxidectins requires epidemiologically appropriate and sustainable measures.
- As a consequence, (targeted) selective anthelmintic treatment is a much-needed, rational, and therefore highly valuable deworming approach, especially for adult horses.
- This method has been successfully used in several countries and many horse owners show a high degree of compliance.

INTRODUCTION

Parasites are an integral part of the global fauna, and consequently parasitic infections are ubiquitous in horses. Parasitism represents a significant consideration for any appropriate horse breeding, husbandry, and management program. However, when properly managed, equine parasite infections rarely pose major problems or can be successfully handled and treated. The authors present the most relevant horse helminths with an emphasis on temperate areas, in a priority ranking—according to pathogenic potential and the horse's age—and propose ways of keeping these infections under control by applying evidence-based medicine. Conventional interval treatment

Dedication: In memory of Prof. Gene Lyons, an outstanding equine parasitologist.
[a] Parasite Consulting GmbH, Wendschatzstrasse 8, CH-3006 Berne, Switzerland; [b] Institute of Comp. Tropical Medicine and Parasitology, LMU – University Munich, Munich, Germany; [c] Department of Infectious Diseases and Immunology, Faculty of Vet. Medicine, Utrecht University, Yalelaan 1, 3584CL Utrecht, The Netherlands
* Corresponding author. Institute of Comp. Tropical Medicine and Parasitology, LMU – University Munich, Munich, Germany.
E-mail address: kpfister@duc.ch

Vet Clin Equine 34 (2018) 141–153
https://doi.org/10.1016/j.cveq.2017.11.009
0749-0739/18/© 2017 Elsevier Inc. All rights reserved.

measures that have led to the development of significant drug resistance are contrasted with a more efficacious and highly targeted antiparasitic approach.

PARASITE SPECIES IN ORDER OF PATHOGENICITY
Parascaris spp

Horses ingest the thick-walled *Parascaris* eggs while grazing. The eggs hatch and larvae begin to migrate from the intestine, through the liver to the lungs (about 1–2 weeks after infection). Subsequently, larvae penetrate the alveolar capillaries to enter the airways, and migrate via the bronchi to the trachea, are coughed up and swallowed. Within 3 weeks, larvae are back in the small intestine and develop into adult worms. The prepatent period is approximately 9 to 16 weeks. Elimination of all eggs from the environment (stables, paddocks, pastures) is virtually impossible; larvated eggs can survive for years.

STRONGYLES ("LARGE" AND "SMALL" STRONGYLES)
Large Strongyles (Strongylus spp.)

The 3 species of this genus (*Strongylus vulgaris*, *S edentatus*, and *S equinus*) are robust, dark-red nematodes (10–50 mm) residing in the cecum and colon, and undergoing mandatory, parenteral migration in their larval stages. *Strongylus* spp. infections are pasture-associated parasite infections and on pasture, the excreted eggs develop into infective larvae 3 (L3). Ingested L3 undertake a parenteral migration and subsequent development occurs outside the alimentary tract.

S vulgaris larvae migrate along arteries and congregate at the root of the cranial mesentery artery, where they remain for several months and undergo a molt to L5 before returning to the large intestine via circulation. *S vulgaris* adults begin to lay eggs approximately 6 to 7 months after infection. In many parts of Europe and North America, *S vulgaris* has become rare.

S edentatus larvae move via portal veins to the liver and migrate through the parenchyma before further migrating beneath the peritoneum of the ventral abdomen and flanks and returning to the intestinal lumen. The prepatent period of *S edentatus* is approximately 11 months.

After first forming nodules in the gut wall, *S equinus* larvae also travel to the liver to migrate through the parenchyma before continuing to the pancreas and returning to the large intestine; the prepatent period is approximately 8 to 9 months.

Small Strongyles (Cyathostomins)

Small strongyles encompass more than 50 species, of which about 10 comprise more than 98% of all small strongyle populations. These nematodes (4–25 mm) reside exclusively in the cecum and colon, and may be present in huge numbers, often exceeding 100,000 per horse. The prevalence of small strongyles in young (<4 years), pastured horses approaches 100%, so cyathostomin infections are virtually ubiquitous in grazing horses. Despite their high prevalence, adult cyathostomins generally do not inflict pathology. Owing to similarities of morphology, biology, and epidemiology, these nematodes are usually considered as a single entity, and therefore are discussed accordingly.

Eggs produced by adult cyathostomins develop into infective L3s on the pasture in the presence of appropriate climatic conditions. After ingestion, L3s invade the gut wall and are enclosed in a fibrous capsule of host origin (encysted stages). After intervals ranging from weeks to perhaps more than 2 years, larvae emerge into the intestinal lumen and molt into young adult worms. The prepatent periods vary from 5 weeks to several months, depending on species and whether larvae undergo arrested development while in the host. Favorable microclimatic conditions on pastures during the grazing season not only facilitate the hatching of eggs and the development to infective stages, but also the survival of L3s for extended periods. These conditions all contribute to accumulation of infective larvae on pastures toward the end of the grazing season, posing an increased risk of infection. In temperate climates, infective L3s can overwinter on the pasture, especially if protected by a snow cover, and be a source of reinfection in the spring.

Anoplocephala and Anoplocephaloides

All cestodes (tapeworms) require an intermediate host; for equine tapeworms, these hosts are oribatids (mites), which are ubiquitous in forage and associated soils. Thus, tapeworm infections are most frequent in pasture-based management systems. Three species of tapeworms are known to equids. *Anoplocephala perfoliata*, 2.5 to 4 cm, is the most common, and is predominantly found in the cecum near the ileocecal junction. *A magna* (up to 50 cm) and *Anoplocephaloides* (1–4 cm) are usually found in the small intestine. Equids are infected while grazing and ingesting oribatid mites with an infective metacestode stage. After a prepatent period of at least 6 weeks, adult worms produce thick-shelled, irregularly round- or trapezoidal-shaped eggs containing an oncosphere surrounded by a pear-shaped apparatus. Mite populations amplify similar environmental conditions also favorable for strongylid larval development, so there seems to be an increased risk for horses during late summer and autumn.

Other intestinal parasitic infections include *Strongyloides westeri*, *Trichostrongylus axei*, *Oxyurids*, *Cryptosporidium* spp. (in foals), *Giardia* spp. (in foals), and *Gasterophilus* spp. Three bot species, *G intestinalis*, *G nasalis*, and *G haemorrhoidalis*, have been introduced into the Americas. All these species should be specifically diagnosed and treated according to available drugs and published recommendations.

CLINICAL SIGNS IN VARIOUS AGE GROUPS

Virtually every horse harbors some intestinal parasites, beginning at a few days of age and continuing throughout its life. The majority of these infections cause no clinical signs, either because the parasite is inherently nonpathogenic, or is not present in sufficient numbers to disrupt homeostasis. Regardless, any abnormal clinical signs of the alimentary tract should trigger some consideration for parasitic disease, even in horses that recently received anthelmintic treatment.

This article's scheme for addressing clinical parasitoses is (i) to rank horses into distinct age groups, (ii) to identify distinct clinical signs, and (iii) to formulate a differential diagnostic list of potential parasitic pathogens.

New-Born Foals up to Weaning

Alimentary clinical signs

Diarrhea at 2 to 3 weeks of age could be associated with the protozoa *Cryptosporidium* spp. or occasionally by *S westeri*. These infections can be accompanied by inappetence, diarrhea, unthriftiness, and emaciation.

Foals are susceptible to *S westeri* infections until about 6 months of age. *S westeri* mainly reside in the duodenum and jejunum, and may cause local mucosa erosions followed by inflammation and edema. When present in large numbers, the infection can lead to catarrhal enteritis and diarrhea; clinical signs may be associated with high *Strongyloides* egg counts. Diarrhea in young foals may be caused by different circumstances (eg, postfoaling estrus of the mare), the presence of *Strongyloides* eggs in a foal with diarrhea is not proof of cause and effect.

Developing stages of *Cryptosporidium* spp. in the lower part of the small intestinal mucosa are responsible for stunting and swelling of microvilli. Severe infections can be accompanied by watery diarrhea.

Parascaris spp. are the most common pathogenic parasites of foals. Potential clinical signs include diarrhea, obstipation and/or colic, lethargy, rough coat, pot-bellied appearance, and weight loss or poor growth. Adult *Parascaris* reside in the small intestine, and worst case scenarios can involve intestinal obstruction or impaction, with potential intestinal perforation and fatal peritonitis. Ascarid impactions frequently occur within 48 hours after deworming the foal with anthelmintics that have a neuromuscular mode of activity (eg, avermectins, moxidectins, and pyrantel).

Low burdens of adult *Parascaris* generally remain asymptomatic. *Parascaris* disease mainly occurs during the first year of life, because strong protective immunity develops, independent of treatment.

Weaned Foals from 6 to 12 Months of Age

Alimentary clinical signs

Until the onset of protective immunity, *Parascaris* infections can cause diarrhea, impaction colic, and unthriftiness. Large *Parascaris* burdens can contribute to mechanical obstruction of the intestinal lumen.

This age group of foals may exhibit colic caused by either *Parascaris* spp. or migrating *S vulgaris* larvae, resulting in proliferative endarteritis with potential thromboembolic sequelae, obstruction of the mesenteric circulation, and intestinal infarction.

Diarrhea and unthriftiness in foals have been associated with emerging larval stages of cyathostomins.

Anoplocephala infections occasionally are the cause of alimentary signs related to ileal obstruction or cecal intussusceptions. They can be very difficult to diagnose definitively ante mortem.

Juveniles 1 to 4 Years of Age

Alimentary clinical signs

Adult small and large strongyles, even when present in high numbers, generally do not cause alimentary signs, mainly because they reside in the gut lumen and do little damage to the intestinal mucosa. Adult worms are observed occasionally in the feces, but they provide no indication of the size of the worm burden or their pathogenicity.

As part of their obligatory life cycle, larval cyathostomins invade the mucosa and submucosa of the cecum and colon, causing inflammation marked by edema, hemorrhage, and accumulation of eosinophilic and mononuclear cells. The severity of mucosal lesions varies with the number of ingested larvae and the immune status of the host. Burdens of several hundred thousand worms are not uncommon. The most severe syndrome associated with small strongyle infection results from mass emergence of large numbers of encysted cyathostomin larvae. Such emergence usually coincides with the cessation of arrested development, which explains its late winter or early spring seasonality in northern temperate climates. This syndrome, termed larval cyathostominosis, may also be triggered by a recent anthelmintic treatment during seasons when high numbers of hypobiotic larvae have accumulated. Removal of luminal worm populations by deworming may stimulate the emergence of encysted larvae to repopulate the vacated niche.

Clinical signs of larval cyathostominosis include watery diarrhea, dramatic weight loss, and ventral edema. Horses suffering from larval cyathostominosis exhibit hypoalbuminemia, hyper-β-globulinemia, a decreased albumin to globulin ratio, leukocytosis, dehydration, and additional physiologic disruptions. Larval cyathostominosis cannot be reversed by therapeutic deworming, and severe cases have a high mortality rate.

Diarrhea, colic, and unthriftiness may also be associated with *Anoplocephala* infections, presumably related to ulceration of the cecal mucosa at their attachment sites. This may lead to ileal impaction, cecal intussusception, and spasmodic colic.

Nonspecific or general clinical signs

Migrating larvae of *S vulgaris* cause proliferative endarteritis and thrombus formation in juvenile horses, as well as in foals. Pathologic changes within the circulatory system include aneurysm and thromboembolic infarction. The major clinical sign is colic.

Tail rubbing is a common response to pruritus of the perianal region, caused by the egg-laying activity of adult *Oxyuris*. Pinworm infection is not restricted to any age category, although historically younger horses were more prone to infection. Local skin infections and damage to the hair coat are the major consequences of pinworm infection.

Although *Parascaris* eggs can still be detected in juvenile horses, severe clinical signs are no longer expected.

Adult Horses (>4 Years of Age)

Alimentary clinical signs

In general, parasites cause minimal clinical disease in mature horses, so specific diagnostic measures are recommended rather than rote, empirical deworming.

Larval cyathostominosis may occur in adult horses subsequent to massive larval exposure or compromised immunity. *Parascaris* eggs are occasionally detected in the feces of mature horses, but clinical signs are not expected.

Other parasitic causes of unthriftiness or colic in adult horses include *Anoplocephala* infections and larval *S vulgaris* infections.

DIAGNOSTIC PROCEDURES

Clinical signs, age, and a recent deworming history are undoubtedly insufficient to arrive at a definitive parasitologic diagnosis. Clinical decisions should always be substantiated by laboratory diagnostics. Many procedures can be performed in a veterinary practice setting with appropriately trained and supervised staff and requires minimal specialized equipment.

Merely detecting the presence of reproductive products is sufficient to confirm some tentative diagnoses. For example, demonstration of *Oxyuris* eggs in a perianal scraping is sufficient to confirm a diagnosis of oxyurosis in a tail rubbing horse. In contrast, strongyle eggs are so ubiquitous in the feces of grazing horses that their mere presence does not confirm strongylosis as the cause of the present signs.

CONTROL OF PREVALENT GASTROINTESTINAL PARASITES

This section focuses on Strongyles (large and small strongyles), *Parascaris* and *Anoplocephala* and presents a modern, sustainable program called selective anthelmintic treatment (SAT) in comparison with the conventional interval dose treatment.

CONVENTIONAL INTERVAL TREATMENT

The introduction of the benzimidazoles in the 1960s was soon followed by a novel approach to parasite control, that is, using anthelmintics to disrupt the life cycle of horse nematodes. This treatment approach consisted of repeated deworming at regular intervals, which effectively coincided with the egg reappearance period of common strongylid nematodes. This regimen, termed the interval dose system, was developed by Drudge and Lyons,[1] and its main objective was control, if not eradication, of S vulgaris. A rote regimen of bimonthly or 3 to 4 times per year deworming rapidly supplanted targeted treatments based on a specific diagnosis. Regrettably, routine habit displaced monitoring for efficacy, and undoubtedly contributed to the ubiquity of benzimidazole resistance. As other anthelmintic classes became available for commercial use, the same schedules were followed and the inevitable consequence was resistance in other target parasites as well, most notably Parascaris spp.[2,3]

The basic element responsible for the success of the interval system was deworming at a frequency coincident with the egg reappearance period of the target parasite(s).[4] The various anthelmintic classes have different egg reappearance periods, (https://aaep.org/guidelines/parasite-control-guidelines) and deworming at intervals equal to or shorter than the egg reappearance period can select very intensively for anthelmintic resistance (AR).

Blind treatments (those administered without specific diagnostic evidence) against Anoplocephala traditionally consisted of 1 or 2 anthelmintic treatments against cestodes with either praziquantel or pyrantel during the spring and/or autumn. Based on tapeworm epidemiology, a single-blind treatment in the autumn is acceptable if Anoplocephala is known to be endemic on a farm.

Performing diagnostics to know when to treat for Parascaris is more difficult, because heavy infections can rarely cause problems during larval migration, and treatments against adult worms can cause intestinal blockage in foals and weanlings.

Blind treatments with any dewormer should not be administered unless the AR status of the herd is known. Use of anthelmintics against resistant populations is clinically ineffective, and contributes to further intensification of the resistance status. Establishing the resistance status of endemic Parascaris strains is critical, because macrocyclic lactone resistance is ubiquitous, and pyrantel resistance has been documented in several herds.

ANTHELMINTIC RESISTANCE

AR is the ability of parasites to survive dosages of drugs that were effective against the same species and stage of infection when the product was first introduced.

The universal use of benzimidazoles since the mid-1960s resulted in highly prevalent resistance among cyathostomins by the late 1970s. Resistance against the tetrahydropyrimidines exists in many parts of the world, and at least in North America may be related to the availability of formulations for daily dosing in the United States and Canada.[5] Resistance of cyathostomins to both of these drug classes now occurs worldwide.[2,6]

It was hypothesized that AR to macrocyclic lactones would not develop readily in cyathostomins or Parascaris, owing to the presence of large environmental refugia (the proportion of the parasite population not under selection pressure of an anthelmintic, here, pasture L3s and embryonated eggs). Resistant Parascaris spp. were first reported by Boersema and colleagues,[3] but since in many countries.[7,8]

During recent decades, the macrocyclic lactones have been used mainly or exclusively on many premises, and in many intensively managed facilities the control of cyathostomins was done through blind anthelmintic treatments, without monitoring for AR.

Pursuing alternative strategies to slow the development of macrocyclic lactone resistance in cyathostomins should be a priority, because no classes of anthelmintics with new modes of action are currently under development for horses.

HOW TO DETECT RESISTANCE

Fecal egg count reduction testing (FECRT) is still considered the gold standard for detecting AR in vivo. Nevertheless, it may be difficult to document true AR among cyathostomins, especially if FECRT indicates that the anthelmintic is still highly effective against the adult stages.[9]

Because more than 50 species of cyathostomins have been identified, it seems probable that various species have differing susceptibilities to AR development.[10] Lyons and colleagues[11] found luminal larval stages shortly after ivermectin treatment in necropsied horses and suggested that these larval stages had survived owing to macrocyclic lactone resistance. A shortened egg reappearance period may indicate the development of macrocyclic lactone resistance in larval stages.[12]

Fortunately, many authors have published on the interpretation of equine parasitologic diagnostics, and recent guidelines for interpreting equine FECRTs in a research setting have been adopted in the United States.[5] Owing to reported shortening of the egg reappearance period on some premises,[13] egg counts for FECRT comparisons should not be limited to days 0 and 14, but should also be performed at 42 or 56 days after treatment with ivermectin or moxidectin, respectively.

A critical analysis of various issues associated with conventional interval treatment clearly demonstrates that more appropriate monitoring and alternative control regimens are needed.[5,14,15] Also, it is, in the author's opinion, unnecessary and ecologically and ethically inappropriate to treat a high percentage of horses that do not show any detectable gastrointestinal parasite infection.

THE NOVEL CONTROL PROGRAM "SELECTIVE ANTHELMINTIC TREATMENT" STRATEGY IN CONTRAST WITH THE "CONVENTIONAL INTERVAL DOSE TREATMENT" OR ("ROTE DEWORMING STRATEGY")

The SAT deworming strategy focuses on the presence of strongyles as an essential prerequisite for treatment. With the SAT approach, only horses with individual egg counts of 200 eggs per gram of feces (EpG) or higher will be treated with anthelmintics. Alternatively, groups of horses, with a maximum of 10 animals in a pool, would be treated as a group when the average strongyle egg count exceeds 100 EpG. An additional consideration for modifications to SAT would be the documented presence of other, potentially pathogenic parasites. For additional background information for Northern European countries, with mild climatic conditions see the following websites: "Decision Tree Horse" (http://www.parasietenwijzer.nl/eng/horse/GB_DesicionTreeHorse.html) or "Cavallo – Calendar" (http://www.cavallo.de/pferde-medizin/wurmkur-fuers-pferd-selektive-entwurmung-und-weidehygiene.626691.233219.htm#1, or for North America: https://aaep.org/sites/default/files/Guidelines/AAEPParasiteControlGuidelines_0).

SELECTIVE ANTHELMINTIC TREATMENT AND REFUGIA

SAT is a valuable, alternative anthelmintic approach that has been adopted rapidly in several areas of Europe and North America. In Denmark, this system has even been mandated by national regulation. At present, use of the SAT system is restricted to adult horses, although some promising results have been reported for horses less than 3 years of age.[16]

The SAT system is based on the distribution of intestinal worms within a host population. It is well-known that the majority of parasites occur in a limited number of individuals within any host population.[17,18] Accordingly, only some adult horses are wormy, although up to 50% of all herd members shed very few or no worm eggs in the feces.[19] This "low shedding" proportion requires few if any anthelmintic treatments.[20–22]

Some readers will misconstrue selective treatment as an attempt to deworm only those individuals with high worm burdens. However, it should be noted that the magnitude of a horse's worm burden cannot be quantified ante mortem and alternative criteria for treatment selection must be considered. Although egg counts are not correlated with worm numbers, strongyle egg shedding is a good indicator of future infection pressure on contaminated pastures, and high-contaminating horses often shed more eggs than the rest of the herd combined. When low- or zero-shedders are sorted out on a particular farm, fecal monitoring and anthelmintic treatments can be concentrated on the high egg shedders, who are responsible for the majority of contamination. An international consortium of equine parasitologists has set a tentative threshold for a strongyle treatment at 200 EpG (IEIDC meeting Kentucky 2012).

How does one implement a SAT program for a given horse population?

- Three fecal samples should be examined from each herd member during the first year as a baseline and characterization of the horses in a herd. All horses repeatedly shedding 200 EpG or more are characterized as high strongyle egg shedders, and will consequently be treated regularly, in contrast with other members of the herd.
- All horses with an egg count higher than the threshold will be appropriately dewormed with a product known to be effective against the target strongyle population.
- Regardless of their egg counts, individual horses that seem to demonstrate clinical manifestations of a parasitic disease may be specifically dewormed on the recommendation of a veterinarian.
- Because anthelmintic treatment is limited to horses shedding high numbers of worm eggs, contamination of the horse paddocks and pastures will be significantly reduced over time.
- This method will allow for a simultaneous efficacy evaluation of the drugs administered. To monitor AR development, fecal samples for quantitative examination should be collected before treatment, at Day 14 and again 42 days after ivermectin treatment, and 56 days after dosing with moxidectin. For anthelmintics containing benzimidazoles or pyrantel salts, fecal counts should be performed at 14 days after treatment. FECRT is conducted to compare changes in egg counts presumably owing to anthelmintic treatment.
- Detection of AR within the herd will drive decisions regarding anthelmintic selection, and can help to prevent spreading of resistant strains on the pastures and paddocks.
- Low and/or moderate contaminator horses (egg counts below threshold level of 200 EpG) will continue to shed eggs without any selection pressure, and thereby contribute positively to the maintenance of *refugia* on the pastures.
- Continuous egg shedding by low EpG horses may enhance host immunity through constant stimulation of host defense factors.
- The SAT system provides adequate parasite management for horse herds, while promoting and maintaining controllable *refugia*.[23]

The SAT system can be modified for individual horses or for characterized groups of horses for premises with very large populations of equids.

SELECTIVE ANTHELMINTIC TREATMENT PRACTICAL TREATMENT PROCEDURE
General Considerations

Owing to the ubiquity of AR in cyathostomins and ascarids, it is recommended that no antiparasitic treatments should be administered to adult horses without preceding diagnostics. In some countries, such as Denmark, prophylactic anthelmintic treatment is forbidden by law.

A comprehensive diagnostic analysis, at least at the herd level, would include a (pooled) larval culture or a molecular-based analysis to demonstrate the presence or absence of large strongyles on the farm. Because up to 50% of adult horses within a discrete population may shed no or very few nematode eggs, there is no medical indication for the anthelmintic treatment of those individuals, let alone of the entire herd. It is recommended that comprehensive records of fecal examinations be maintained, because historical evidence could support future changes to the parasite management program.

After examining 3 samples from each horse during the introductory year, horses can be classified confidently as low, moderate, or high egg shedders. Egg counts from individual horses are very repeatable,[21,22,24] so future monitoring could be performed at a lower frequency.

Although initial monitoring makes parasite control more demanding than rote treatment programs, these measures are justifiable from a veterinary medical and ethical point of view. Moreover, selective treatment uses fewer doses of drugs, with evident economic and ecologic advantages.

On premises that still have endemic *S vulgaris* populations, it is recommended to administer a moxidectin treatment to all horses during late autumn (mid-November to mid-December). The objective of such a treatment is to reduce the number of migrating large strongyle larvae, plus a portion of encysted cyathostomin larvae, with the added benefit of concurrently removing *Gasterophilus* spp instars over wintering within the horse.

For any specific anthelmintic treatment, it is essential to know the resistance status for that drug class in the resident parasite population. Also, the egg reappearance period after the use of that drug on the farm should be compared with the published egg reappearance period at the time of initial introduction. A shortened egg reappearance period may be a sign of developing resistance. SAT can only be successful if AR testing is an integral feature of the program.

ADULT HORSES
Single Horses and Small Groups

The SAT system can be adopted for single horses or very small herds. After characterizing the contamination potential of the horse(s) with 3 samples during the first grazing season, treatment decisions are implemented as for larger groups. Thereafter, a treatment schedule may be followed as outlined in the "Cavallo-Calendar" or the "Decision tree" or the American Association of Equine Practitioners guidelines. A horse that never exceeds the threshold level of 200 EpG will not require any treatment, but should be monitored in the future with at least 1 fecal analysis per year. Horses with strongyle EpG of 200 or greater, or with diagnostic evidence of *Parascaris* or cestode infections should be treated and/or monitored according to the "Cavallo – Calendar" (http://www.cavallo. de/pferde-medizin/wurmkur-fuers-pferd-selektive-entwurmung-und-weidehygiene. 626691.233219.htm#1), or "Decision Tree"(http://www.parasietenwijzer.nl/eng/horse/ GB_DesicionTreeHorse.html), or the American Association of Equine Practitioners guidelines (https://aaep.org/sites/default/files/Guidelines/AAEPParasiteControlGuidelines_0).

If products other than macrocyclic lactones remain efficacious against strongyles, they should be used preferentially, and macrocyclic lactones be kept in reserve. If *S vulgaris* is detected, either through larval cultures or by polymerase chain reaction, it is recommended that the entire group be treated with a macrocyclic lactone.

If *Parascaris* is present, however, the horse should not be treated with macrocyclic lactones unless the AR status on the farm has been determined. For *Anoplocephala*, the drugs of choice are either praziquantel or a double dose (13.2 mg/kg) of pyrantel. Nematocides and cestocides can be combined if there is a simultaneous need for treatment of small strongyles. In general, however, combination products should not be used unless there is specific evidence of concurrent nematode and cestode infections.

Horses in Large Populations

SAT can be implemented for large herds of horses as previously. However, modifications may be considered if age-clustered groups of horses are regularly kept together on the same pasture. In such cases, fecal samples from subgroups of horses (eg, n = 10) can be pooled, and the threshold for treating such a group is 100 EpG for strongyles.[25] Detection of *Parascaris* eggs, however, will require that—out of a positive pooled sample—individual fecal samples be examined to identify the affected horse(s). Thereafter, the same schedules can be followed as for individual horses. Thus, treat individual horse if eggs of *Parascaris* are detected, and treat the whole herd if eggs from *Anoplocephala* are detectable.

For optimal epidemiologic benefit, all horses on a single premise should participate in a SAT system, particularly any that share a common grazing venue.

Geriatric Horses

Opinions vary whether geriatric horses are more susceptible to parasitic disease. However, fecal analyses are highly recommended for geriatric horses with compromised health, followed by anthelmintic treatment if appropriate.

HORSES AT BREEDING FARMS

Mares and stallions at breeding facilities may be managed the same way as other adult horses with the SAT system. However, owing to the high economic value of breeding animals, owners and managers may be much more reluctant to "trust" selective treatment, and may prefer to maintain an interval treatment program, or even to administer pyrantel tartrate on a daily basis.

In North America, pyrantel tartrate is approved for daily administration (2.64 mg/kg/d) and the aim is to prevent the establishment of immature strongyles or ascarids after the ingestion of infective stages. Daily pyrantel tartrate has label claims against large strongyle adults (*S vulgaris*, *S edentatus*, and *Triodontophorus* spp.), cyathostomin adults, and fourth stage larvae, *Oxyuris equi* adults and fourth stage larvae, and *Parascaris equorum* adults and fourth stage larvae. Daily pyrantel tartrate can, under certain circumstances, be a very useful management tool. One example would be individual treatment of high-shedding horses that graze with a herd. By reducing the fecal egg count of a selected number of horses, the potential exposure for the entire group is reduced. But, application to entire groups of horses is rarely necessary because low and moderate shedders may not cause sufficient contamination to justify the expense, and this tenet applies to all individual anthelmintic treatments of low to moderate shedding horses.

There is a reasonable concern that daily exposure of a parasite population to an anthelmintic compound would help to select for resistance. However, pyrantel tartrate has no activity against encysted mucosal or migrating larval stages, so a considerable proportion of the worm burden of horses on daily treatment is technically *in refugia* (a worm population that is not subjected to a pharmaceutical drug, eg, parasite stages on the pasture, etc). Horses maintained on daily pyrantel tartrate still produce strongyle eggs, albeit in fewer numbers than if they were not on this prophylactic program.[26]

TREATMENT AND PREVENTION OF *GASTEROPHILUS* INFESTATIONS

In areas with endemic *Gasterophilosis*, a treatment for larval stages is indicated even though these parasites are generally of low pathogenicity. In the Northern hemisphere, it is recommended that all horses on farms at risk be treated during late autumn, after pasture grazing has terminated and adult flies are no longer active. Owing to the broad spectrum of the macrocyclic lactones, the only efficacious drug class, a specific treatment for *Gasterophilus* spp. effectively serves as a so-called late fall treatment against large strongyles and/or larval cyathostomins.

TREATMENT OF *ANOPLOCEPHALA* INFECTIONS

Anoplocephala infections should be targeted with a single active ingredient, unless there is diagnostic evidence of concurrent nematode and cestode infections. Unfortunately, praziquantel is not available as a single treatment option in every country. Because *Anoplocephala* is endemic in most herds, and these infections are very difficult to detect, all horses in a given herd should be treated whenever positive diagnoses are made in individual horses. Because *Anoplocephala* populations accumulate over the grazing period, it is recommended to administer a single treatment near the end of summer to reduce worm burdens through the winter.[27]

INFECTION POTENTIAL IN STABLES

The biological development of strongyles from eggs to the infective L3 stage is strongly associated with vegetation on pastures, that is, grazing, climate, humidity, and so on. Although some limited larval development may also occur in stables or even on bare ground or paddocks, the contribution of these larvae to the total uptake for horses is quantitatively irrelevant.

Foals can also acquire infective roundworm eggs or *S westeri* larvae in a stable. Therefore, hygienic measures should be implemented.

Last, horses of all ages can acquire *Oxyuris* infections when stabled.

PASTURE INFECTIONS AND PASTURE MANAGEMENT

Because pastures are the major, immediate source of strongyle and tapeworm infections, pasture management plans should consider the potential impact of any measures on transmission of these parasites. As shown by Herd,[28] frequent removal of feces from horse pastures (2–3 times weekly, depending on the climate) affords significant reduction of pasture infectivity, thereby reducing the potential of reinfection for grazing horses.

However, such labor-intensive measures are rarely implemented, owing to lack of staff or equipment. Certain alternative strategies have been considered.

1. It has been shown repeatedly that "cross-grazing" of horses with sheep or cattle can significantly reduce pasture larval transmission.[29]

2. Rotational grazing can be very effective, but proper implementation requires a thorough understanding of parasite epidemiology in the local area. Strongyle larvae can survive for long intervals on pasture under the right environmental conditions, and tend to accumulate over a grazing season. Contaminated pastures often remain infective even in the absence of horses.

ACKNOWLEDGMENTS

The authors sincerely thank Dr Craig R. Reinemeyer, Rockwood, Tennessee, for his greatly appreciated editorial help, his constructive and critical comments, and his frankness toward our ideas.

REFERENCES

1. Drudge JH, Lyons ET. Control of internal parasites of the horse. J Am Vet Med Assoc 1966;148:378–83.
2. Boersema JH, Borgsteede FHM, Eysker M, et al. The prevalence of anthelmintic resistance of horse strongyles in The Netherlands. Vet Q 1991;13:209–17.
3. Boersema JH, Eysker M, Nas JW. Apparent resistance of Parascaris equorum to macrocyclic lactones. Vet Rec 2002;150:279–81.
4. Reinecke RK. Chemotherapy in the control of helminthiasis. Vet Parasitol 1980;6: 255–92.
5. Kaplan RM. Anthelmintic resistance in nematodes of horses. Vet Res 2002;33: 491–507.
6. Chapman MR, French DD, Monahan CM, et al. Identification and characterization of a pyrantel pamoate resistant cyathostome population. Vet Parasitol 1996;66: 205–12.
7. Hearn FPD, Peregrine AS. Identification of foals infected with Parascaris equorum apparently resistant to ivermectin. J Am Vet Med Assoc 2003;223:482–5.
8. Stoneham S, Coles GC. Ivermectin resistance in Parascaris equorum. Vet Rec 2006;158:572.
9. Coles GC, Bauer C, Borgsteede FH, et al. World Association for the Advancement of Veterinary Parasitology (W.A.A.V.P.) methods for the detection of anthelmintic resistance in nematodes of veterinary importance. Vet Parasitol 1992;44: 35–44.
10. van Doorn DCK, Ploeger HW, Eysker M, et al. Cylicocyclus species predominate during shortened egg reappearance period in horses after treatment with ivermectin and moxidectin. Vet Parasitol 2014;206:246–52.
11. Lyons ET, Tolliver SC, Collins SS. Probable reason why small strongyle EPG counts are returning "early" after ivermectin treatment of horses on a farm in Central Kentucky. Parasitol Res 2009;104:569–74.
12. Lyons ET, Tolliver SC. Further indication of lowered activity of ivermectin on immature small strongyles in the intestinal lumen of horses on a farm in Central Kentucky. Parasitol Res 2013;112(2):889–91.
13. Geurden T, van Doorn, Claerebout D, et al. Decreased egg re-appearance period after treatment with ivermectin and moxidectin in horses in Belgium, Italy and the Netherlands. Vet Parasitol 2014;204:291–6.
14. Nielsen MK, Pfister K, von Samson-Himmelstjerna G. Selective therapy in equine parasite control—Application and limitations. Vet Parasitol 2014;202(3):95–103.
15. Pfister K, Scheuerle M, van Doorn D, et al. Insights, experiences and scientific findings of a successful worm control in several European countries and the perspectives for the future. J Equine Vet Sci 2016;39:S45–6.

16. Schnerr CU. Feldstudie zur Epidemiologie und Bekämpfung von Strongyliden in Pferdebeständen im Raum Baden-Württemberg (Doctoral dissertation, LMU-Munich). 2011.
17. Anderson RM, May RM. Population dynamics of human helminth infections: control by chemotherapy. Nature 1982;297:557–63.
18. Schneider S, Pfister K, Becher A, et al. Strongyle infections and parasite control strategies in German horses – a risk assessment. BMC Vet Res 2014;10:262–76.
19. Comer KC, Hillyer MH, Coles GC. Anthelmintic use and resistance on thoroughbred training yards in the UK. Vet Rec 2006;158:596–8.
20. Becher AM, Mahling M, Nielsen MK, et al. Selective anthelmintic therapy of horses in the Federal states of Bavaria (Germany) and Salzburg (Austria): an investigation into strongyle egg shedding consistency. Vet Parasitol 2010;15:116–22.
21. Döpfer D, Kerssens CM, Meijer YGM, et al. Shedding consistency of strongyletype eggs in Dutch boarding horses. Vet Parasitol 2004;124:249–58.
22. Nielsen MK, Haaning N, Olsen SN. Strongyle egg shedding consistency in horses on farms using selective therapy in Denmark. Vet Parasitol 2006;135:333–5.
23. van Wyk JA. Refugia-overlooked as perhaps the most potent factor concerning the development of anthelmintic resistance. Onderstepoort J Vet Res 2001;68: 55–67.
24. Scheuerle MC, Stear MJ, Honeder A, et al. Repeatability of strongyle egg counts in naturally infected horses. Vet Parasitol 2016;228:103–7.
25. Eysker M, Bakker J, van de Berg M, et al. The use of age-clustered pooled faecal samples for monitoring worm control in horses. Vet Parasitol 2008;151:249–55.
26. Reinemeyer CR, Prado JC, Andersen UV, et al. Effects of daily pyrantel tartrate on parasitologic and performance parameters of young horses repeatedly infected with cyathostomins and *Strongylus vulgaris*. Vet Parasitol 2014;204:229–37.
27. Roelfstra L, Betschart B, Pfister K. A study on the seasonal epidemiology of Anoplocephala spp.-infection in horses and the appropriate treatment using a praziquantel gel (Droncit 9% oral gel). Berl Munch Tierarztl Wochenschr 2005;119: 312–5.
28. Herd RP. Epidemiology and control of equine strongylosis at Newmarket. Equine Vet J 1986;18(6):447–52.
29. Eysker M, Jansen J, Mirck MH. Control of strongylosis in horses by alternate grazing of horses and sheep and some aspects of the epidemiology of Strongylidae infections. Vet Parasitol 1986;19:103–15.

Practical Fluid Therapy and Treatment Modalities for Field Conditions for Horses and Foals with Gastrointestinal Problems

C. Langdon Fielding, DVM

KEYWORDS

- Intravenous fluids • Pain management • Antimicrobials • Oral fluids • Hypovolemia
- Colic

KEY POINTS

- Fluid therapy should use both the oral and the intravenous route when possible, but a functioning gastrointestinal system is required to effectively use oral fluids.
- Fluid therapy (oral or intravenous) can be administered by bolus or continuous infusion, and each method has specific advantages and disadvantages.
- Pain management is an essential aspect of field treatment and should be initiated early and allow for additional diagnostic testing and treatments to be completed.
- In neonatal foals, antimicrobial coverage may be appropriate in most, if not all, cases of gastrointestinal disease.
- In older animals, greater than 2 to 3 months of age, routine antimicrobial use for gastrointestinal disease should be avoided unless a specific bacterial focus exists that is likely to respond to antimicrobial administration.

INTRODUCTION

In many equine practices, there is increasing demand for higher levels of diagnostic testing and treatment services in the field. Point-of-care laboratory testing, ultrasound machines, and endoscopy and radiography systems all have portable options. In many instances, a diagnosis can be made without ever leaving the farm. Similar expectations for treatment also exist, and ambulatory practitioners should be familiar with the options and controversies surrounding the field management of the horse or foal with gastrointestinal (GI) disease.

The author has nothing to disclose nor any conflicts of interest.
Loomis Basin Equine Medical Center, 2973 Penryn Road, Penryn, CA 95663, USA
E-mail address: langdonfielding@yahoo.com

There are many practical considerations for the field treatment of GI disease, but this article focuses on 3 areas whereby the field practitioner will often be required to make decisions:

1. Fluid therapy
2. Pain management
3. Antimicrobials

Although these same concepts apply to the management of horses in both hospital and field conditions, there are some unique considerations in the field that must be addressed. The major limitation in the field is often the availability of facilities and personnel. Rapid fluid administration can be challenging without appropriate height for hanging fluids, and catheters can easily be damaged or dislodged in stalls that are not appropriate for horses receiving intensive care. Safety of the personnel handling the horse is important and affected by adequate pain control in horses that are rolling or repeatedly getting up and down. The decision for antimicrobial use is often made without the benefit of complete laboratory testing results. Despite these limitations, field treatment has benefits, including familiar surroundings for the horse and more rapid initiation of treatment. The remainder of this article examines these 3 main areas of consideration when initiating field treatment of GI diseases in horses and foals.

SECTION 1: FLUID THERAPY

The need for fluid therapy in the field will often be determined using a combination of the following:

1. Physical examination findings
2. Historical information
3. Owner preferences

Physical Examination Findings

Some of the simplest physical examination findings of dehydration can be easily evaluated:

1. Prolonged skin tenting
2. Dry/tacky mucous membranes
3. Urine concentration

However, recognition of dehydration using clinical examination findings is unreliable.[1,2] Even with increased experience and training, clinicians are often unable to accurately quantify the degree of dehydration. The clinical signs of hypovolemia/hypoperfusion may be easier to detect as compared with those of dehydration. Although these are rarely used to determine an exact amount of fluid loss (or volume needed for replacement), they are excellent markers to suggest that fluid therapy is warranted:

1. Heart rate
2. Pulse quality
3. Mucous membrane color
4. Capillary refill time
5. Mentation
6. Extremity temperature
7. Jugular refill time
8. Urine output

When multiple perfusion parameters are abnormal, fluid therapy is likely to be warranted. However, similar to dehydration parameters, fluid therapy should not be based on these examination findings alone. In many cases, even when referral to a hospital is planned, some degree of stabilization with fluids before transport is indicated.

Historical Information

Historical factors that may influence the decision to begin fluid therapy include the duration of illness, decreased water intake (if noted by owner), or excessive fluid losses (sweating, diarrhea, and so forth). A history of chronic nonsteroidal anti-inflammatory drug (NSAID) use or previous episode of renal failure may also influence decisions about fluid therapy. Given the limitations of the physical examination to accurately detect dehydration, these historical factors are often important in decision making.

Owner Preferences

Finally, owner preferences may play a large role in the decision to initiate fluid therapy in the field. An owner may have had a previous sick animal that they perceived was saved by fluid treatment in the field or conversely an animal that was lost in transport because they thought treatment was delayed. There may be financial reasons for postponing treatment or refusing hospital or referral care.

Ultimately, the recommendation to initiate fluid therapy in the field should first be made based on the clinical examination and historical factors on an individual case basis. However, consideration of the facilities and personnel available as well as the owner preferences must also be taken into account. A treatment plan that considers all of these factors will be most likely to lead to success and owner satisfaction, as opposed to forcing a plan that is not practical or not desired by the client. When owners elect field treatment instead of hospital referral, equine practitioners should carefully note this decision in the medical record.

Once the decision has been made to begin fluid therapy, there are 2 main choices that must be made:

1. Enteral and/or intravenous (IV) administration of fluids
2. Bolus or continuous administration of fluids

Enteral Versus Intravenous Fluid Administration

There have been several excellent research studies evaluating the benefits of enteral fluids to treat many forms of equine GI disease.[3-6] However, a near universal requirement for this mode of treatment is a functioning GI system that can manage and use enteral fluid administration. Although this concept seems incredibly simple, the importance of a functional GI tract cannot be emphasized enough.

The presence of significant net gastric reflux (>4 mL/kg) would be an indication that enteral fluid therapy may not be effective or even detrimental. However, the lack of net reflux when a nasogastric tube is placed does not guarantee that the horse will tolerate significant volumes of enteral fluids. It is not uncommon to administer enteral fluids to a horse without net reflux, only to return hours later and find a similar volume of fluid waiting in the stomach when a nasogastric tube is placed again. Such fluids would have had limited beneficial effect for the horse.

Indications that enteral fluid therapy may not be appropriate:

a. Net gastric reflux >4 mL/kg
b. Disease process likely to be associated with ileus
c. Ultrasound examination consistent with ileus or gastric distention (**Fig. 1**)

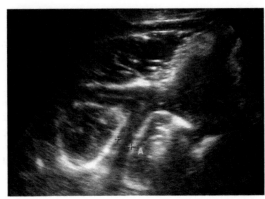

Fig. 1. Ultrasound image of small intestine in a horse with signs of colic. This small intestine may be unable to effectively absorb water from the oral administration of fluids.

IV fluids effectively bypass the GI system, and this attribute can be both an advantage and a disadvantage. In a horse with a poor ability to absorb enteral fluid, IV fluids can be life saving. However, conditions in which high fluid volumes are desired within the GI system (ie, impactions), IV fluids may be less effective than enterally administered fluids.[3–5] IV fluids typically take a longer time to administer than enteral fluids (particularly in bolus administration), and this is another important factor to consider for treatment in the field.

Most equine practitioners carry only one type of IV fluid on their truck in the larger 3- to 5-L bags that are appropriate for horses. Ideally, this fluid would be appropriate for as many different types of equine emergencies as possible. For equine GI disease, an isotonic crystalloid is usually appropriate, and the author prefers one of the commercially available acetated fluids (**Table 1**). These fluids typically have a lower chloride concentration than lactated Ringer solutions or 0.9% saline solution, which may be advantageous.[7] Hypertonic saline (7.2%) is also used in critical cases of equine GI disease, but should be followed with an isotonic IV fluid.

An important point to note, a combination of IV and enteral fluid administration is appropriate in horses with a functioning GI system. Conversely, in horses with enteritis and/or reflux, IV fluids should be used alone.

Enteral Versus Intravenous Fluid Administration in Foals

The author's practice frequently manages foals with GI disease in the field with IV fluid therapy. Enteral fluid therapy in foals is common in patients that are not able to nurse; however, this is used less frequently as a primary means for hydrating neonatal

Table 1					
Common crystalloid fluids used in the field					
Fluid	**Na$^+$ (meq/L)**	**K$^+$ (meq/L)**	**Cl$^-$ (meq/L)**	**Ca^{++} (meq/L)**	**Mg^{++} (meq/L)**
Normosol R	140	5	98	0	3
Lactated Ringer solution	130	4	109	3	0
0.9% Saline	154	0	154	0	0
7.2% Saline (hypertonic)	1232	—	1232	—	—

patients with GI disease. In neonatal foals, the GI system is often not functioning, the cost of IV fluids is minimal, and the time for administration of IV fluids is short. For all of these reasons, the IV route may be preferred over the oral route.

Bolus Versus Continuous Infusion of Fluids

After deciding whether to use the oral or IV route for fluid administration, the practitioner must next decide the rate of administration. Bolus administration has 2 distinct advantages:

1. Hypovolemia/dehydration is corrected more rapidly.
2. Less time is required for administering fluids.

Continuous fluid infusion (or smaller intermittent bolus administration over a prolonged period of time) could be less likely to cause fluid overload and may be more effective in rehydrating the animal. However, it will be slower to correct hypovolemia and will require more of the practitioner's time.

A. Practical recommendations for the *bolus* administration of IV fluids to a moderately dehydrated/hypovolemic horse include the following:
   1. Use a 12- to 14-gauge IV catheter (larger catheters may have a higher rate of complications)[8]
   2. Use large-bore IV sets[9]
   3. Raise the fluids as high as possible if trying to achieve rapid rates
   4. Use a volume of 20 to 40 mL/kg bolus of an isotonic crystalloid over 1 to 2 hours
B. Practical recommendations for the *bolus* administration of enteral fluids to a moderately dehydrated/hypovolemic horse would include the following:
   1. 10 to 15 mL/kg bolus of water through a nasogastric tube
   2. Electrolytes may be added to the administered fluids
   3. Larger volumes are possible, but more conservative amounts may prevent associated signs of colic
   4. An additional 10 to 15 mL/kg bolus can be administered every 30 to 60 minutes if the horse is tolerating the enteral fluids well

There are many options for the electrolyte composition of enterally administered fluids. The following combination has been recommended to create an enteral fluid that is similar to the electrolyte concentrations in equine plasma and has been safe to administer to horses in large volumes[10]:

1. 5.27 g/L of NaCl
2. 0.37 g/L of KCl
3. 3.78 g/L of $NaHCO_3$

As a practical approximation, a practitioner could start with a 10-L bucket of drinking water, add 50 g of NaCl (regular table salt), 4 g of KCl (a sodium-free salt alternative), and 40 g of $NaHCO_3$ (baking soda) and create an appropriate fluid for administration.

Many variations of this combination are possible. Fluids with a very low sodium concentration should not be repeatedly administered in large volumes because hyponatremia may develop.

C. Practical recommendations for the *continuous* infusion of IV fluids to a moderately dehydrated/hypovolemic horse include the following:
   1. 2 to 4 mL/kg/h of an isotonic crystalloid is typically appropriate for patients without significant ongoing losses.

2. Patients with significant volumes of diarrhea or reflux can require as much as 10 mL/kg/h of an isotonic crystalloid.
3. Fluid rate should be set at: Ongoing losses/h (L/h) + 2 mL/kg/h = Administered rate (L/h)

D. Practical recommendations for the *continuous* infusion of oral fluids to a moderately dehydrated/hypovolemic horse include the following:

1. 2 to 4 mL/kg/h of oral electrolyte solution
2. Fluids can be dosed intermittently every 1 to 2 hours

Bolus Versus Continuous Intravenous Fluids in the Field Treatment of Foals

Foals with GI disease are often treated with initial bolus fluid administration (20 mL/kg) of an acetated, isotonic IV crystalloid because this can be a very practical and effective means to stabilize these hypovolemic patients. The author finds continuous administration of IV fluids to foals in the field to be quite challenging particularly with inexperienced clients. Smaller volume (eg, 10 mL/kg) fluid boluses can be repeated every 3 to 6 hours, depending on the amount of fluids being lost (ie, diarrhea or reflux) and the volume of milk that the foal is ingesting. Fluid balance is critically important in foals, and clients and practitioners should carefully monitor for signs of fluid overload with repeated fluid bolus administration.

SECTION 2: PAIN MANAGEMENT IN THE FIELD FOR HORSES WITH GASTROINTESTINAL DISEASE

Pain control is essential for effective field management of GI disease. Without adequate pain management, fluid therapy and diagnostic testing can be extremely difficult to carry out in a horse that is trying to roll or lay down. Many cases of equine GI disease are referred to hospital facilities because of an inability to adequately control the patient's discomfort as opposed to a specific requirement for surgery. In the author's opinion, the immediate cessation of pain is one of the single most important contributions that a veterinarian can make on arrival to evaluate and treat a horse with GI disease. With analgesia, the horse is more easily handled and the owners quickly feel that the situation is under control.

Numerous treatments for pain management are available to the equine practitioner in the field setting, and some of the more common options are discussed later. Similar to fluid therapy, pain management options can be separated into both intermittent and continuous dosing. Some practical notes about the use of continuous infusions in the field should be considered:

1. Pain medications can be added to the bags of IV fluids, but it is important that dosing is calculated carefully and the rate of administration is tightly controlled. Changes in fluid rate will also affect changes in medication administration rate!
2. If owners are assisting with fluid administration wherein medications are included, very detailed instructions are required and the risks need to be explained.
3. Owners should have clear instructions to stop all fluids if the horse's behavior changes or if they have concerns.
4. Infusions can also be given through infusion pumps, but the costs and training to use these devices may make them impractical in many field situations.

If adding continuous pain medications to the IV fluids, the following should be followed:

1. Divide the size of the IV fluid bag (ie, 5 L) by the number of liters per hour (ie, 1 L/h) to get the number of hours per bag.

2. Take the dose of pain medications (ie, 7 mg/h) and multiply by the number of hours per bag to get the number of mg of medication per bag.
3. Example:
   a. Fluid rate of 2.5 L/h
   b. 5-L IV fluid bags
   c. Detomidine rate of 0.01 mg/kg/h (5 mg/h to 500-kg horse)
   d. Add 10 mg detomidine per 5-L bag of fluids
   e. IMPORTANT TO REMEMBER: If the fluid rate changes, so will the rate of medication administration

Nonsteroidal Anti-Inflammatory Drugs

Nonsteroidal anti-inflammatory medications (NSAIDs) are used very commonly in cases of equine GI disease. In some instances, before the arrival of the veterinarian, the owner may have administered these medications. These medications have many reported advantages and disadvantages[11–13] (**Table 2**).

Each case of GI disease should be considered individually when considering whether to administer an NSAID at the start of treatment. Unless there is specific knowledge of renal disease or severe dehydration, a half to full-labeled dose of an NSAID administered to horses exhibiting pain associated with GI disease is a reasonable treatment protocol. IV administration will provide more immediate relief, but oral administration is an option as well. Two frequently used NSAIDs for horses with GI disease include the following:

1. Flunixin meglumine (0.5–1.0 mg/kg)
2. Firocoxib (0.1–0.2 mg/kg)

Firocoxib may be preferred in cases with small intestinal ischemic injury.[14] The use of NSAIDs in neonatal foals with GI disease should be carefully considered. Renal function may already be compromised in these patients, and the chronic administration of flunixin meglumine has been associated with gastric ulceration in foals.[15] However, pain management in foals with enteritis can often be achieved with low doses of flunixin meglumine (0.25 mg/kg IV). In the author's opinion, there are selected cases wherein this class of medications can be appropriate to resolve discomfort while other treatments are initiated.

Alpha-2 Agonists

Alpha-2 agonists are commonly used to provide both pain relief and sedation for horses with GI disease. They are often considered for use when rectal examinations and nasogastric intubation will be performed, because they can help to prevent injury to the horse, handler, and veterinarian. However, the analgesic effects of these medications are significant and should not be underestimated[16] (**Table 3**).

Table 2	
Selected advantages and disadvantages of nonsteroidal anti-inflammatory medications in horses	
Advantages	**Disadvantages**
Rapid administration	Nephrotoxic
Moderate time to onset of pain relief	Association with gastric ulcers
Long duration of action	Association with right dorsal colitis
Anti-inflammatory effects	Long duration of action
Reasonable cost	

Three alpha-2 agonists that are available to most equine practitioners are often at the following doses for a single dose administration:

1. Xylazine (0.2–1 mg/kg IV)
2. Romifidine (0.04 mg/kg IV)
3. Detomidine (0.01 mg/kg IV)

The negative effects of alpha-2 agonists in horses with GI disease are frequently emphasized, including inhibition of GI motility and gastric emptying.[17,18] Some practitioners also feel that these medications may mask the animal's true degree of pain, thereby potentially delaying surgery. However, the ability to immediately halt signs of discomfort and provide safety for those handling the horse makes these drugs invaluable.

The alpha-2 agonists can be used as intermittent bolus medications or as continuous infusions. Intermittent bolus administration is a safe way to administer this class of drugs because it allows the veterinarian to observe the horse as each dose wears off. Improvement or deterioration in clinical signs can be evaluated and additional doses considered at each time point.

Continuous infusions are appealing because they smooth out the "ups and downs" associated with intermittent bolus administrations. Client satisfaction is often higher with continuous infusions, but it can be difficult to assess changes in the horse's condition. In the author's experience, intermittent bolus injections are best used at the beginning of treatment and during the evaluation period. Once a treatment plan has been decided (ie, management at the farm instead of referral), continuous infusions can be used to provide relief to the horse and owner while treatment continues. It is extremely important that the veterinarian takes the time to educate the owner on the clinical signs indicating that the infusion dose is too high or low.

Detomidine can be a particularly effective drug to use as a continuous infusion to manage painful horses that do not require surgery or do not have a surgical option. The author has used continuous infusions over a 12-hour period to provide relief to horses with GI pain while waiting for the beneficial effects of rehydration and time. In cases where there is not a definitive need for euthanasia and surgery is not indicated, an infusion of this medication can be invaluable to relieve suffering and provide comfort to the owner. Infusion doses of 2 alpha-2 agonists for use in horses are the following:

1. Detomidine: 0.01 to 0.02 mg/kg/h
2. Xylazine: 0.5 to 1.5 mg/kg/h

An initial bolus dose of the medication can be given before starting the infusion (see dosages above).

In addition to IV bolus administration and continuous infusions, alpha-2 agonists can also be given intramuscularly (IM). Detomidine can be used IM for longer-term pain

Table 3	
Selected advantages and disadvantages of alpha-2 agonist medications in horses	
Advantages	**Disadvantages**
Rapid administration	Inhibit GI motility
Rapid onset of pain relief	Short duration of action
Short duration of action	Induction of diuresis
Reasonable cost	

management but the effects will be less pronounced than IV administration.[19] Dose titration will be easier with IV administration or infusion, however.

The author has not used continuous infusions of alpha-2 agonists in neonatal foals. These medications can provide profound analgesia and sedation in foals, but cardio-vascular and respiratory depression can also be significant.

Opioids

Opioids represent an additional class of analgesic medication that can be used for field management of pain in equine GI disease. There continues to be debate about the visceral analgesia provided by opioids in horses.[20,21] Butorphanol is an agonist-antagonist opioid analgesic that is often used in combination with alpha-2 agonists. Similar to the alpha-2 agonists, its primary use can be sedation for completion of procedures or for pain control (**Table 4**).

Butorphanol can be administered as intermittent bolus doses or as a continuous infusion.[22] Butorphanol is often given as an initial IV bolus dose (0.01–0.02 mg/kg) for procedures in the field combined with alpha-2 agonists. If continuous pain control is needed, an infusion (0.013 mg/kg/h) can be started and has several benefits over intermittent bolus dosing, including smoother pain control and decreased negative effects of the medication.[22] Intermittent bolus administration of butorphanol can be given IV or IM.

Butorphanol (0.05 mg/kg IV) has been shown to have analgesic effects in healthy foals.[23] The author typically uses a dose of 0.01 to 0.02 mg/kg of butorphanol IV often combined with midazolam (0.1–0.2 mg/kg IV) in foals. There is less information available regarding its use in sick foals. The author has not used continuous infusions of butorphanol in neonatal foals.

Lidocaine

Lidocaine is a class 1B sodium channel blocker. Lidocaine has several potential benefits that directly relate to the management of GI disease in horses (**Table 5**).[24,25]

Lidocaine is typically administered with a loading dose of 1.3 mg/kg, followed by a continuous infusion of 0.05 mg/kg/min (3 mg/kg/h). Some practices do not use the loading dose and simply begin the infusion recognizing that there will be a longer time to reach steady state and the full effect of the infusion. Lidocaine has some additional benefits in that it may diminish some of the negative effects of NSAIDs on the GI system.[26] For this reason, the author incorporates lidocaine in pain management for GI disease whenever it is practical. The author does not use lidocaine as commonly for field management, because it requires continuous infusion and the analgesic effects may be inadequate for horses with more severe discomfort. In addition, side effects are not uncommon and may be difficult for owners to recognize.

To the author's knowledge, lidocaine infusions have not been evaluated in neonatal foals. However, the author has used these infusions (2–3 mg/kg/h) in foals

Table 4	
Selected advantages and disadvantages of opioid medications in horses	
Advantages	**Disadvantages**
Rapid administration	Inhibit GI motility
Rapid onset of pain relief	May cause excitation at high doses
Moderate duration of action	Analgesia and sedation may be milder compared with other
Reasonable cost	medications

Table 5	
Selected advantages and disadvantages of lidocaine use in horses	
Advantages	**Disadvantages**
Minimal inhibition of GI motility	Used primarily as a continuous infusion
Reasonable cost	Can cause ataxia or recumbency if given too quickly
Anti-inflammatory	
Analgesic	

with enteritis in a hospital setting. Close supervision is required to use these infusions with foals in the field, because an accidental bolus administration could be life threatening.

SECTION 3: ANTIMICROBIAL USE IN THE FIELD FOR HORSES AND FOALS WITH GASTROINTESTINAL DISEASE

The third major category of therapeutics for consideration in field management of GI cases is the use of antimicrobials for horses with GI disease. For the purposes of this article, foals (less than 2–3 months of age) will be considered separately because the disease conditions and negative effects of antimicrobial administration are different between these age groups.

Antimicrobial Use in Horses with Gastrointestinal Disease that Are greater than 2 to 3 months of Age

The decision to initiate antimicrobial therapy in horses over 2 to 3 months of age with suspected GI disease is complex. Abdominal sepsis is one of the major indications for antimicrobial use. This can be due to septic peritonitis, which can often be associated with an internal abscess or GI perforation. Infectious enteritis caused by specific bacteria such as *Neorickettsia risticii*, *Rhodococcus equi*, *Lawsonia intracellularis*, *Clostridium difficile*, or *Clostridium perfringens* are additional indications for early initiation of antimicrobial therapy.[27] However, there are other causes of enteritis such as equine coronavirus, salmonellosis, and other undiagnosed causes that are less likely to benefit from antimicrobial therapy. Antimicrobial therapy itself can cause GI disease through changes in the GI microbiome.[28]

In cases of enteritis, concerns over bacterial translocation are often considered an additional reason for antimicrobial treatment whereby there may be intestinal inflammation and compromise of the mucosal barrier. A low white cell count (specifically a low neutrophil count) may also be considered an indication for antimicrobial use in this patient population.

When evaluating the evidence for the use of antimicrobials in adult horses with GI disease (other than septic peritonitis), it is difficult to find strong support for this practice.[29] Studies have shown the presence of bacteremia in some horses with colitis; however, a similar investigation into horses with colic is warranted.[30] Previous treatment with antimicrobials does not affect the incidence of bacteremia.[30] Likewise, the presence of bacteremia does not necessarily mean that antimicrobials will reduce later complications associated with infections.

Even more importantly, there is evidence that antimicrobial use is associated with the development of colitis due to *C difficile*.[28] Given the potentially negative effects of antimicrobial administration and the lack of proven beneficial effects, the author thinks that these medications should be restricted to cases in which a suspected and/or proven infection is likely to respond to antimicrobials. Diagnosis of a specific pathogen is unlikely to take place on the first visit to the farm, and therefore, antimicrobial use at initial treatment of adult horses is not routinely indicated unless there is a high suspicion for a specific bacterial focus. As further research is completed, these recommendations may change for specific diseases. Likewise, if septic complications (ie, septic thrombophlebitis) develop, then appropriate antimicrobial use would be warranted.

Foals

Antimicrobial use in neonatal foals with GI disease has many similar considerations as in adult horses. However, there is less evidence of negative effects of antimicrobial use on the GI system of newborn foals. In addition, bacteremia and subsequent septic foci are more frequently identified in newborn foals (joints, lungs, umbilical structures) than in adult horses.

A clinical trial evaluating routine antimicrobial coverage for foals with a variety of GI disease (meconium impaction, enteritis, and so forth) is greatly needed. Until such time, it is prudent to continue to cover these patients with broad-spectrum antimicrobials to minimize the chances for sepsis secondary to GI disease. However, continued consideration of responsible antimicrobial stewardship is important.

OTHER MEDICATIONS FOR FIELD MANAGEMENT OF GASTROINTESTINAL DISEASE IN HORSES

Numerous medications can be considered for the management of a wide variety of GI diseases in horses. This article focuses on 3 key areas of decision making for the equine field practitioner. Treatments for gastric ulceration are considered in Pilar Camacho-Luna and colleagues' article, "Advances in Diagnostics and Treatments in Horses and Foals with Gastric and Duodenal Ulcers," in this issue. Although not specifically fitting into the 3 categories of this article, N-butylscopolammonium bromide (0.3 mg/kg IV or IM) can be an effective addition to field management of the horse with GI disease. This medication can decrease the signs of colic in many horses, but may not be effective for horses with more severe clinical signs.

CLINICAL PROTOCOLS FOR FIELD MANAGEMENT OF EQUINE GASTROINTESTINAL DISEASE
Example 1: Prolonged and Significant Gastric Reflux (>4 mL/kg/h)

Horses can develop intestinal ileus with infectious enteritis, peritonitis, exercise-associated exhaustion, or for unknown reasons. Regardless of the cause, horses with ileus often have extensive and ongoing fluid losses, abdominal discomfort, and a GI system that is unlikely to handle oral fluid administration.

Practical plan for field management:

1. IV fluid administration of an isotonic crystalloid
   a. Fluid rate = Rate of gastric reflux (L/h) + 2 to 4 mL/kg/h
2. Additional supplementation of dextrose (1 mg/kg/min) in the IV fluids if prolonged anorexia is present (over 24–48 hours in adult horses; immediately in neonatal foals)
3. Placement of nasogastric tube to remove and quantify reflux
4. Administration of NSAID initially if well hydrated
5. Administration of an initial bolus dose of alpha-2 agonist to facilitate nasogastric intubation and to control pain
6. Continuous infusion of lidocaine to manage pain

Example 2: Prolonged and Significant Diarrhea

Horses can develop diarrhea for a variety of causes, and many do not require extensive management if the horse is eating and drinking normally. However, in cases with dehydration or anorexia, field treatment can be very effective. Causes of infectious diarrhea include *Salmonella*, *Clostridia* sp, and *Neorecketsia risticii*. Sand ingestion and other noninfectious causes of diarrhea may also require field treatment.

Practical plan for field management:

1. IV fluid administration of an isotonic crystalloid
   a. Fluid rate = Approximate estimate of diarrhea (L/h) + 2 to 4 mL/kg/h
2. Administration of NSAID initially if well hydrated
3. Administration of an initial bolus dose of alpha-2 agonist and butorphanol to facilitate diagnostic procedures and to control pain
4. Continuous infusion of lidocaine to manage pain (if needed)
5. Continuous infusion of butorphanol to manage pain (if needed)
6. Continuous infusion of alpha-2 agonist to manage pain (if needed)

Example 3: Impaction Colic with Mild Abdominal Discomfort

Feed impactions of the large colon are commonly described in horses and can frequently be treated in the field. More severe cases that have surgical treatment options should be referred to a facility where abdominal surgery can be performed if required. Impactions of the small colon and other intestinal segments can also develop, and many may be managed in the field as well depending on the specifics of the case.

Practical plan for field management:

1. Oral fluid administration through a nasogastric tube only if net reflux is not present: Initial bolus of 15 mL/kg followed by repeat administration of 8 mL/kg every 30 to 60 minutes
2. IV fluid administration of an isotonic crystalloid
   a. Fluid rate = 2 to 4 mL/kg/h
3. Administration of NSAID initially if well hydrated
4. Administration of an initial bolus dose of alpha-2 agonist and butorphanol to facilitate diagnostic procedures and to control pain
5. Continuous infusion of lidocaine to manage pain (if needed)
6. Continuous infusion of alpha-2 agonist to manage pain (if needed)

Example 4: Gas Distended and Severely Painful Colic

Severe gas distention can develop with many different types of colic, including ileus, feed obstructions, and strangulating lesions. Initial pain control is important, but field management should be considered after evaluation of the owner's willingness to pursue surgery or more intensive care at a hospital facility.

Practical plan for field management:

1. Oral fluid administration through a nasogastric tube only if net reflux is not present: Initial bolus of 16 mL/kg followed by repeat administration of 8 mL/kg every 30 to 60 minutes
2. IV fluid administration of an isotonic crystalloid
   a. Initial fluid bolus 20 to 40 mL/kg
   b. Continuous fluid rate = 2 to 4 mL/kg/h
3. Administration of NSAID initially if well hydrated

4. Administration of an initial bolus dose of an alpha-2 agonist and butorphanol to facilitate diagnostic procedures and to control pain
5. Continuous infusion of alpha-2 agonist to manage pain (if needed and referral/surgery is not an option)

REFERENCES

1. Vega RM, Avner JR. A prospective study of the usefulness of clinical and laboratory parameters for predicting percentage of dehydration in children. Pediatr Emerg Care 1997;13:179–82.
2. Pritchard JC, Burn CC, Barr AR, et al. Validity of indicators of dehydration in working horses: a longitudinal study of changes in skin tent duration, mucous membrane dryness and drinking behaviour. Equine Vet J 2008;40:558–64.
3. Lopes MA, White NA 2nd, Donaldson L, et al. Effects of enteral and intravenous fluid therapy, magnesium sulfate, and sodium sulfate on colonic contents and feces in horses. Am J Vet Res 2004;65:695–704.
4. Lopes MA, Walker BL, White NA 2nd, et al. Treatments to promote colonic hydration: enteral fluid therapy versus intravenous fluid therapy and magnesium sulphate. Equine Vet J 2002;34:505–9.
5. Hallowell GD. Retrospective study assessing efficacy of treatment of large colonic impactions. Equine Vet J 2008;40:411–3.
6. Lester GD, Merritt AM, Kuck HV, et al. Systemic, renal, and colonic effects of intravenous and enteral rehydration in horses. J Vet Intern Med 2013;27:554–66.
7. Fielding L. Crystalloid and colloid therapy. Vet Clin North Am Equine Pract 2014; 30:415–25.
8. Higgins J. Preparation supplies and catheterization. In: Fielding CL, Magdesian KG, editors. Equine fluid therapy. 1st edition. Hoboken (NJ): Wiley-Blackwell; 2015. p. 129–41.
9. Nolen-Walston RD. Flow rates of large animal fluid delivery systems used for high-volume crystalloid resuscitation. J Vet Emerg Crit Care (San Antonio) 2012;22:661–5.
10. Lopes MA. Enteral fluid therapy. In: Fielding CL, Magdesian KG, editors. Equine fluid therapy. 1st edition. Hoboken (NJ): Wiley-Blackwell; 2015. p. 261–78.
11. Marshall JF, Blikslager AT. The effect of nonsteroidal anti-inflammatory drugs on the equine intestine. Equine Vet J Suppl 2011;39:140–4.
12. McConnico RS, Morgan TW, Williams CC, et al. Pathophysiologic effects of phenylbutazone on the right dorsal colon in horses. Am J Vet Res 2008;69:1496–505.
13. Holland B, Fogle C, Blikslager AT, et al. Pharmacokinetics and pharmacodynamics of three formulations of firocoxib in healthy horses. J Vet Pharmacol Ther 2015;38:249–56.
14. Cook VL, Meyer CT, Campbell NB, et al. Effect of firocoxib or flunixin meglumine on recovery of ischemic-injured equine jejunum. Am J Vet Res 2009;70: 992–1000.
15. Traub-Dargatz JL, Bertone JJ, Gould DH, et al. Chronic flunixin meglumine therapy in foals. Am J Vet Res 1988;49:7–12.
16. Roger T, Ruckebusch Y. Colonic alpha 2-adrenoceptor-mediated responses in the pony. J Vet Pharmacol Ther 1987;10:310–8.
17. Sutton DG, Preston T, Christley RM, et al. The effects of xylazine, detomidine, acepromazine and butorphanol on equine solid phase gastric emptying rate. Equine Vet J 2002;34:486–92.

18. Zullian C, Menozzi A, Pozzoli C, et al. Effects of α2-adrenergic drugs on small intestinal motility in the horse: an in vitro study. Vet J 2011;187:342–6.

19. Mama KR, Grimsrud K, Snell T, et al. Plasma concentrations, behavioural and physiological effects following intravenous and intramuscular detomidine in horses. Equine Vet J 2009;41:772–7.

20. Sanchez LC, Robertson SA, Maxwell LK, et al. Effect of fentanyl on visceral and somatic nociception in conscious horses. J Vet Intern Med 2007;21:1067–75.

21. Muir WW, Robertson JT. Visceral analgesia: effects of xylazine, butorphanol, meperidine, and pentazocine in horses. Am J Vet Res 1985;46:2081–4.

22. Sellon DC, Roberts MC, Blikslager AT, et al. Effects of continuous rate intravenous infusion of butorphanol on physiologic and outcome variables in horses after celiotomy. J Vet Intern Med 2004;18:555–63.

23. McGowan KT, Elfenbein JR, Robertson SA, et al. Effect of butorphanol on thermal nociceptive threshold in healthy pony foals. Equine Vet J 2013;45:503–6.

24. Peiró JR, Barnabé PA, Cadioli FA, et al. Effects of lidocaine infusion during experimental endotoxemia in horses. J Vet Intern Med 2010;24:940–8.

25. Robertson SA, Sanchez LC, Merritt AM, et al. Effect of systemic lidocaine on visceral and somatic nociception in conscious horses. Equine Vet J 2005;37:122–7.

26. Cook VL, Jones Shults J, McDowell MR, et al. Anti-inflammatory effects of intravenously administered lidocaine hydrochloride on ischemia-injured jejunum in horses. Am J Vet Res 2009;70:1259–68.

27. Uzal FA, Diab SS. Gastritis, enteritis, and colitis in horses. Vet Clin North Am Equine Pract 2015;31:337–58.

28. Båverud V, Gustafsson A, Franklin A, et al. Clostridium difficile: prevalence in horses and environment, and antimicrobial susceptibility. Equine Vet J 2003;35:465–71.

29. Dunkel B, Johns IC. Antimicrobial use in critically ill horses. J Vet Emerg Crit Care (San Antonio) 2015;25:89–100.

30. Johns I, Tennent-Brown B, Schaer BD, et al. Blood culture status in mature horses with diarrhoea: a possible association with survival. Equine Vet J 2009;41:160–4.

Enteral/Parenteral Nutrition in Foals and Adult Horses Practical Guidelines for the Practitioner

Elizabeth A. Carr, DVM, PhD

KEYWORDS

- Enteral nutrition • parenteral nutrition • Equine • Critical illness

KEY POINTS

- The metabolic response to starvation in healthy individuals includes a decrease in metabolic rate and sparing of body proteins.
- The catabolic response to injury or inflammation may increase metabolic rate and protein breakdown despite a decrease in nutritional intake.
- Enteral nutrition provides intraluminal nutrition to the gut and can improve gut barrier integrity, mass, protein content, motility, and function.
- Parenteral nutrition provides nutritional support when the enteral route is unavailable.
- Parenteral nutrition must be handled with strict aseptic techniques and should be gradually introduced and discontinued to prevent metabolic consequences.

INTRODUCTION
Protein/Calorie Malnutrition

The average, healthy adult horse can apparently tolerate food deprivation (protein/calorie malnutrition [PCM] or simple starvation) for 72 hours with few systemic effects. During the first hours to days of starvation, glycogen stores are used from various tissues (liver, kidney, muscle) for glucose production. As glucose becomes limited, many body tissues begin to rely on fatty acid oxidation and the production of ketone bodies as energy sources. Glycerol produced from lipid degradation, lactate from the Krebs cycle, and amino acids provided from muscle tissue breakdown continue to be used for gluconeogenesis to provide energy to glucose-dependent tissues (central nervous system and red blood cells). This response to starvation correlates with an increase in circulating levels of growth hormone, glucagon, epinephrine, leptin, and cortisol and a

Disclosure Statement: No Disclosures.
Department Large Animal Clinical Sciences, College of Veterinary Medicine, Michigan State University, D202 VMC, 736 Wilson Road, East Lansing, MI 48824-1314, USA
E-mail address: carre@msu.edu

decrease in insulin and thyroid hormones. During PCM, there is an increased drive to eat and a decrease in energy expenditure. Metabolism slows in an effort to conserve body fuels, and the body survives primarily on fat stores, sparing lean tissue until such a time as refeeding occurs.[1]

Although similar adaptive responses to PCM can occur in the healthy older foal, the neonate has limited body reserves. The healthy newborn foal should have enough liver glycogen to support energy needs for several hours of life. However, glycogen stores at birth can vary significantly with illness or prematurity. Lack of nutritional reserves can result in hypoglycemia and hypothermia and quickly affect the ability to maintain normal function and behavior. A weak suck response often develops, leading to an increased risk of aspiration pneumonia, which can start a vicious cycle of deterioration. Consequently, when treating an inappetent neonate, institution of nutritional support is recommended as quickly as possible.

Catabolic Response to Injury

During illness or after trauma, food intake frequently decreases. However, despite this decline in intake, the adaptive responses to starvation do not occur. In contrast to PCM in humans and laboratory animals, the metabolic response to injury (eg, critical illness, sepsis, trauma, surgical manipulation) is characterized by an increased metabolism and the onset of a catabolic process leading to excessive breakdown of tissue proteins, which are used as a metabolic fuel. Insulin resistance develops and hyperglycemia may occur despite the absence of food intake. This metabolic state is the result of a complex interaction of inflammatory cytokines, circulating hormones, and neurotransmitters and is designed to provide endogenous substrates for gluconeogenesis, wound healing, immune cell replication, and synthesis of acute phase.[2] Although this response is beneficial, long-term muscle breakdown results in loss of muscle strength, visceral organ dysfunction secondary to loss of structural and enzymatic proteins, impaired wound healing (caused by loss of precursors for wound healing), immunosuppression, and compromise to the patient's overall health.

Food deprivation during this hypermetabolic/catabolic state results in a much greater loss of lean muscle mass and visceral protein than would be expected during simple starvation.

Nutritional supplementation will reverse the catabolic processes occurring during simple starvation but will not completely reverse those occurring during metabolic stress because as long as tissue injury persists, catabolic processes are maintained. The goals of nutritional support in critical illness should be to save life, maintain muscle mass, preserve and improve cellular and tissue function, and speed recovery.[3] More recently, research in nutritional therapy has focused on attenuating the metabolic response to stress, preventing oxidative cellular injury, and favorably modulating the immune response with the ultimate goals being to reduce disease severity, complications, and length of stay and improve outcome.

The purpose of this article is to review methods and goals for nutritional support of equids in the field, not to make recommendations for treating critically ill patients in an intensive care setting. However, it is worth noting that there continues to be significant debate in human medicine regarding the value of early nutritional support in critical illness.[4–8]

Indications for Nutritional Support

Individuals with pre-existing PCM are at a disadvantage when intake is restricted because of illness. In both humans and laboratory animals, nutritional supplementation has been shown to positively influence both survival and morbidity during critical illness.[9] Nutritional support should be considered in patients with an increased metabolic rate (eg, young growing animals), a history of malnutrition or hypophagia, underlying metabolic abnormalities that could worsen with food deprivation (equine metabolic syndrome, hyperlipidemia), and disorders such as severe trauma, sepsis, burns, or strangulating bowel obstruction that result in an increased energy demand. Underweight horses require nutritional support earlier. Obese or overconditioned individuals, particularly pony breeds; miniature horses and donkeys; individuals with equine Cushing syndrome or equine metabolic syndrome; and pregnant or lactating mares are at risk for hyperlipidemia and should receive nutritional support to try to prevent or minimize hyperlipidemia. If food deprivation is expected to be prolonged, early intervention is indicated to prevent more severe malnutrition.

Routes of Nutritional Support

Although there are conflicting data regarding the pros and cons of parenteral feeding verses enteral feeding, it is clear that enteral feeding has some distinct benefits. Enteral nutrients provide most of the nutrition to the gut and have been shown to improve gut barrier integrity, gut mass, protein content, gut motility, and function in piglets.[10] The complete absence of enteral nutrition results in mucosal atrophy, increased gut permeability, and enzymatic dysfunction in critically ill human patients.[11] Even small amounts of enteral feeding may provide benefits. In a neonatal piglet model, provision of 5% to 10% of nutritional needs by enteral feeding resulted in improved intestinal motility and lactose digestion and decreased mucosal permeability.

The enteral route of nutritional support is simpler, as there is less concern of fluid and electrolyte overload, and this route allows fiber feeding, which cannot be achieved parenterally. Consequently, the enteral route is always preferred when the gastrointestinal tract is functional. However, patients with gastrointestinal disease (inflammation, ileus, or surgical resection) may not be the best candidates for enteral nutrition and may be better off started on parenteral nutrition (PN) while they are gradually reintroduced to enteral nutrition.

Nutritional Requirements

Although the energy requirements of horses of various ages, stages of growth, and activity levels have been determined and equations are available to calculate these needs, the energy and protein requirements for the hospitalized, sick equine patient are not known and likely vary depending on disease state, environment, and level of fitness of the individual. Studies in the human intensive care unit and in sick neonatal foals found that the metabolic energy needs may fall more closely within the range of the resting to maintenance energy requirements of normal, healthy individuals.[9,12,13] The exceptions to this are individuals with extreme trauma, burns or severe sepsis, surgical conditions that require intestinal resection, and large areas of devitalized tissue (eg, clostridial myositis patients that undergo multiple fasciotomy procedures). When estimating the energy requirements of most other equine patients, resting energy requirements are an acceptable target. Resting energy requirements are defined as the amount of energy needed to maintain an individual (no weight gain or loss) in a thermoneutral environment without the metabolic demands of digestion. Maintenance energy requirements include the demands of digestion in this equation and are approximately 30% higher than resting energy requirements. Resting energy requirements vary slightly depending on the size of the horse but can be estimated using approximately 22 to 23 kcal/kg/d for the average full size horse. Maintenance energy requirements can be estimated using 30 to 35 kcal/kg/d. If a patient tolerates nutritional supplementation at resting energy requirements the feeding rate can be gradually increased if needed.

Protein Requirement

The maintenance protein requirement of the healthy adult horse is estimated at approximately 0.5 to 1.5 g/kg/d. The needs of the growing foal are higher and may approach 7 g/kg/d during maximum growth period; additionally, the lysine requirements of growing horses are higher than for mature horses.[13] During critical illness or severe injury, protein catabolism and utilization of amino acids as a source of fuel continue despite the presence of other energy stores. Consequently, when calculating protein requirements in human patients, it is recommended to provide the higher end of the estimated need.[3,14] Another consideration is supplementation of nonessential amino acids that may improve outcome in illness. In humans, glutamine is considered a conditionally essential amino acid and is used as a fuel for enterocytes and other rapidly dividing cells.[15] Glutamine supplementation has been shown to improve clinical outcome in both laboratory and human studies.[16] The amount and ideal route of glutamine supplementation has not been determined in the horse. In one study, glutamine improved mucosal restitution in an oxidant-injured equine colon model.[17] Other recommendations for amino acid supplementation include branched chain amino acids and arginine supplementation. Arginine is a precursor to nitric oxide, is an important vasodilating agent, upregulates immune function and secretion of several hormones, and may reduce ischemia-reperfusion injury.[18,19] Studies looking at specific amino acid supplementation in critically ill or injured horses are currently lacking. Parenteral amino acid solutions that contain nonessential amino acids are available.

Enteral Nutrition

Types of enteral nutrition for adult animals can vary from normal feedstuffs (ie, grains, hay, and complete pelleted diets), slurry diets composed primarily of normal feedstuffs, and liquid diets that allow the clinician to tailor the feeding regimen. In horses with decreased appetite or complete anorexia, the choices are limited to those diets that can be administered through a nasogastric (NG) tube. Complete pelleted feeds offer several advantages—they are relatively inexpensive and well balanced for the maintenance requirements of an adult horse. They contain fiber, which is beneficial for intestinal motility, increasing colonic blood flow, enzymatic activity, and colonic mucosal cell growth and absorption.[20] Disadvantages of pelleted diets lie principally in the difficulty involved in giving them via NG intubation. Powdered commercial diets are now available that provide National Research Council requirements for protein, vitamins, minerals, and fiber. These diets are more easily fed through an NG tube, can be top dressed over normal feedstuffs, can be given by periodic syringe feeding, and have continuous flow through an indwelling small-bore (18F) NG feeding tube (Mila International, Erlanger, KY) or via periodic passage of a NG tube for administration of larger meals. The major disadvantage of these products over complete pelleted diets is their costs.

Both human and equine liquid formulations are available and have been used as enteral nutrition support in horses.[21–25] Alternatively, diets prepared using specific components have been described, although the current availability of powdered diets makes these recipes less useful.[26] Corn oil (or other nonrancid, palatable vegetable oil) may be added to the diet to increase the caloric content but should be added gradually (increasing the intake by one-fourth to one-half cup or 60–120 mL daily not to exceed 2 cups or 500–600 mL total daily intake for a 500-kg horse) to prevent feed refusal and/or diarrhea. Oil should not be added to the ration of hyperlipemic patients. The use of human products (Osmolite and Vital HN) in the mature horse can be very expensive and has been associated with diarrhea and laminitis (although cause and effect are not clear); consequently, they are rarely used and generally not recommended.

Slurry diets made from complete pelleted feeds will not pass through a nasogastric tube using gravity alone. Instead, the slurry should be administered by use of a marine supply bilge pump. If a bilge pump is not available or a large bore tube cannot be passed, pulverizing the pellets before adding water may improve gravity flow. The horse should be checked for the presence of gastric residuals before administration, and the slurry should be pumped slowly with attention paid to the horse's attitude and reaction. The volume of each feeding should not exceed 6 to 8 L per feeding for 450 to 500-kg horses. Studies in healthy horses have found that the feeding of liquid diets is associated with decreased intestinal transit time and decreased prececal starch and fat digestion.[27] Therefore, avoidance of high starch (>25% DE) and high fat (>6% DE) diets is recommended, with the use of highly digestible carbohydrate sources (eg, processed corn starch).

When starting enteral nutrition in a patient with prolonged anorexia, it is recommended to start gradually—the goal is to reach the calculated goal over a period of days. There is no exact formula for the rate of increase or the calculated goal, as many factors (underlying illness, breed, duration of anorexia) will affect the individual's ability to tolerate increased volume enteral feeding. Rapid changes in intake, particularly with component feeding or high-fat diets can be associated with colic or diarrhea. An example of an enteral feeding schedule can be found in **Table 1**.

Enteral Nutrition for Foals

In neonates and young foals, mare's milk is the preferred choice for enteral supplementation. When mare's milk is limited or not available, supplementing with goat's or cow's milk is generally recommended at least through the early neonatal period (first 2 weeks of life). Many neonatologists prefer goat's milk as a better replacement to mare's milk. Although comparison of the fat, protein, and calorie contents of goat, sheep, and cow's milk does not seem to reveal any significant benefit of one over the other, the major whey protein in both goat's and mare's milk is β-lactoglobulin, which may explain the preference, as the major whey protein in cow's milk is α-lactoglobulin.

Gradual transition from one type of milk or replacer is recommended, as rapid changes are often associated with colic, diarrhea, or constipation. If constipation develops, a small amount of mineral oil (5 mL) may be added to tube-fed meals. The fluid characteristics of mineral oil make it unsafe to administer orally, as it will not stimulate a cough reflex if aspirated. Even a small amount of aspirated mineral oil can result in significant pulmonary consolidation and dysfunction.

Long-term supplementation of a foal typically requires switching to milk replacers because of cost and accessibility issues of whole milk products. If using a milk replacer, it is strongly recommended to choose a replacer developed for foals rather

Table 1				
A suggested assisted enteral feeding schedule for a 450-kg horse				
Day 1	**Day 1**	**Day 2**	**Day 3**	**Maintenance (1%–1.5% body weight)**
Number of meals	2–3	3–4	4–6	4–6
Complete feed (kg)/meal	0.5 kg	0.75	0.75–1.0	1.0–1.25
Water (L)/meal	4–6	4–6	6–8	6–8

than an all-species milk replacer. Replacers that contain whey protein are recommended over other protein sources because of digestibility concerns. When feeding milk replacers, it is important to provide a fresh water source, as they are much higher in salt than natural mare's milk, and hypernatremia can develop if a water source is not provided.

Foals normally nurse relatively small amounts of milk frequently throughout the day. When fed larger, less-frequent meals, hunger may cause them to guzzle larger volumes, overloading the small intestinal ability to digest the nutrients resulting in bloating, colic, and diarrhea. Feeding cold milk may help limit large-volume ingestion. An acidified milk replacer is also available; this product is less likely to become rancid when left out for long periods during the warmer season.

Although a healthy, normal foal ingests approximately 15% of its body weight in milk per day during the first few weeks of life (increasing to as much as 30% during the first month), the metabolic demand of a sick, recumbent neonate is likely closer to 5% to 10% (50–100 kcal/kg/d). Before instituting enteral nutrition in a sick foal, it is recommended to assess gastrointestinal motility via abdominal ultrasound scan. Enteral supplementation should be avoided in foals with dilated small intestine or ileus or other signs of enteritis. Small volumes (1%–2% body weight in 24 hours divided into every-2-hour feedings) are recommended when initiating enteral feeding with gradual increase in the volume fed paying careful attention to changes in intestinal motility, gastric residuals, signs of colic, and/or diarrhea. An example of a feeding schedule for a sick neonatal foal can be found in **Box 1**.

Weak, sick foals should be fed by NG tube until strong enough to stand and nurse. If a nurse mare is not available, switching to bucket feeding is ideal to avoid risks of aspiration. When first allowing a foal to nurse, it is often beneficial to milk the mare first and feed the foal via the NG tube. This method decreases the risk of aspiration caused by large-volume let-down by the mare or extreme hunger by the foal. Auscultating their trachea while they nurse can help determine if aspiration is occurring. Once trained to drink from a bucket, the bucket can be hung in the foal's stall, allowing them to drink at will.

Parenteral Nutrition

The major advantage of PN is its ability to supply nutrition when the enteral route is unavailable and to be able to tailor the types of nutrition provided for each individual

---

Box 1
Nutritional plan for sick neonatal foal (50 Kg body weight)

If history of hypoglycemia or inappetence, begin 10% dextrose infusion at ~ 2 mL/min.

Place small NG tube (MILA international). If evaluation suggests foal may tolerate enteral nutrition, start at 1% to 2% body weight/day = 0.5 to 1 L milk/day or ~40 to 80 mL milk q 2 hours.

Check for gastric reflux/residuals before each feeding.

Monitor motility (ultrasound scan, auscultation, palpation) abdominal distension, colic, and diarrhea.

If foal tolerates feedings, can gradually increase volume with initial goal of reaching 5% body weight/day and discontinue intravenous dextrose infusion.

Plan to increase intake to 10% (estimated metabolic requirements of sick)

If foal does not tolerate enteral feeding, discontinue and begin more complete PN (addition of amino acids is critical with lipids to increase calorie intake if necessary).

animal. PN has been found to decrease weight loss, particularly lean body mass, and improve wound healing, immune function, and outcome in human and animal studies when the enteral route cannot be used.[28] In the adult horse, it is most commonly used to supply partial nutrition when oral intake is insufficient or the oral route cannot be used. Individuals that are recumbent or dysphagic, have gastrointestinal disease, or have pre-existing protein/calorie malnutrition should also be considered as candidates for PN.

The major disadvantages of PN are expense and the loss of the beneficial effect of enteral nutrition on maintaining gut function and mass. In humans, the parenteral route may also be associated with an increased risk of infection, although results are contradictory.[28,29] Published reports of PN use in horses primarily consist of case reports with one retrospective evaluating the benefits and risks of PN.[26,30–34]

Formulating Parenteral Nutrition

Depending on the desired goals and duration of supplementation, solutions containing various amounts of carbohydrate, amino acids, lipids, vitamins, electrolytes, and minerals can be formulated. Carbohydrates and lipids are used to meet the horse's energy needs allowing the administered amino acids to be used for wound healing, immune function, and muscle maintenance. Carbohydrate is commonly provided using 50% dextrose solutions. These solutions are hyperosmolar (2525 mOsm/L) and should be infused through a central line or large peripheral vein (jugular vein) to reduce the risk of thrombophlebitis. Lipids are recommended to provide the remainder of nonprotein calories. Lipids are close to isotonic and can be infused separately in a peripheral vein or combined with other components. Lipids come in 10%, 20%, and 30% emulsion and are composed principally of soybean oil (or safflower), egg yolk phospholipids, and glycerin. Lipids should be added to the solution last to avoid destabilization of the emulsion because of an acidic environment. Although recommendations vary, lipids can be added to provide up to 30% to 60% of the nonprotein calories in a PN solution. The addition of lipids to PN is beneficial in patients with persistent hyperglycemia or hypercapnia, reducing the dependency on glucose as the principal energy source. Lipids should be avoided in horses with known hyperlipidemia or in horses suspected of being lipid intolerant. Lipid intolerance can be seen in patients with systemic inflammation, sepsis, or underlying metabolic derangements, and triglyceride levels should be monitored regularly.

Amino acid preparations are available in several concentrations; 8.5% and 10% solutions are most commonly used in veterinary medicine. They are approximately twice the osmolarity of plasma and are acidic and should be mixed with dextrose before adding the lipid component to prevent destabilization of the lipid emulsion. Solutions containing both essential and conditionally essential amino acids, including glutamic acid, would seem to be preferable, although no data on the benefits of conditionally essential amino acids in the sick horses are available. Although there are no clear data on the benefits of a higher protein supplementation, current recommendations in humans are to provide protein in excess of the normal daily requirement because of the higher protein catabolism seen with injury or inflammation. The ratio of nonprotein calories (NPC) to nitrogen should be at least 100:1 in the final solution to limit the use of protein as an energy source (**Boxes 2 and 3**).

Premix solutions are available that contain dextrose and amino acids in varying concentrations. The 2 solutions are separated by a seal that can be broken when ready to use. These products are convenient and can be useful for short-term PN; lipid supplementation is often recommended for longer-term PN.

Box 2
Parenteral nutrition recipe for a neonatal foal

Recipe
1 L 10% Amino Acid solution = 100 g AA	400 kcal
500 mL 50% dextrose solution = 250 g dextrose	850 kcal
500 mL 20% lipid emulsion = 100 g lipids	1000 kcal
Total	2250 kcal/2 L bag
	1.125 kcal/mL

Resting Energy Requirement of sick neonatal foal ~ 45 to 50 kcal/kg/d 50 kg foal needs ~2500 kcal/d to achieve resting energy requirements = 2.2 L/d or ~ 92 mL/h

Provides 110 g protein/day or ~ 2 g/kg body weight. NPC/g nitrogen ration 1850 NPC/17.7 g of nitrogen = 104 (goal is 100–200 NPC/g of nitrogen) Suggested starting rate at 25% resting energy requirements (0.25–0.5 mL/kg/h). Increase rate by 0.25 mL/kg/h every 4–8 hours assuming blood glucose is within acceptable range and no evidence of serum lipemia.

Additional components may be added to PN or given separately including electrolyte solutions and vitamin and mineral supplements. The vitamin and mineral requirements of the critically ill horse are unknown, but published recommendations for healthy horses (NRC 2007) can be used when determining supplementation rates. Based on information in humans, it is strongly recommended to supplement water-soluble B vitamins

---

Box 3
Adult horse parenteral nutrition

PN FORMULATION:

1000 mL 50% dextrose = 500 g dextrose	1700 kcal
1000 mL 10% amino acids (AA) = 100 g AA	400 kcal
500 mL 20% lipids = 100 g lipids	1000 kcal
2.5 L in one bag	3100 kcal/bag

(1 L of 50% dextrose can be purchased in a 2-L bag to allow addition of other components.)
1240 kcal/L or 1.24 kcal/mL

Resting energy requirements

22 to 23 kcal/kg/d

Protein requirements 0.5 to 1.5 g/kg/d:

Example

500-kg horse needs 11,000 kcal/d and 350 g protein

11,000/3100 = 3.5 bags per day or 8 L/d = ~365 mL/h

3.5 bags = 350 g protein
   (Should have 100 to 200 g of NPC/g of nitrogen)

1 g nitrogen = 6.2 g protein

100 g protein/bag = 16.1 g nitrogen

2700 kcal NPC/bag

2700 NPC/16.1 g of nitrogen = 167 (within 100–200 desired)

Suggested starting rate: 25% goal ~100 mL/h. Increase by 100 mL every 4 to 8 hours assuming blood glucose is within acceptable range and no evidence of serum lipemia.

daily, as deficiencies can exacerbate problems associated with refeeding.[35] Although horses synthesize some of the B vitamins in their gastrointestinal tract, chronic inappetence or long-term use of antimicrobials may affect synthesis. Some vitamins are best given orally (vitamins C and E) or added to separate crystalloid solutions (B vitamins). Because fat-soluble vitamins, such as vitamins E, D, and A, are stored in body tissue, they are not generally supplemented unless an individual is off feed for a prolonged period or has an illness that may result in greater use or need. Vitamin E and vitamin A precursors are present in high concentrations in fresh green forage or newly harvested hay. However, the antioxidant benefits of vitamin E may make it worth providing oral supplementation early in illness. Vitamin C is also produced by the horse, and a need for supplementation has not been documented. However, some investigators recommend oral supplementation in sick horses with recommendations of 10 to 20 g per horse per day.[36]

Minerals, if required, are best supplemented in separate crystalloid solutions, as divalent cations may destabilize lipid emulsions. Examples of short-term PN solutions for foals and adults can be found in **Boxes 2** and **3**.

Preparation of PN should be performed under a laminar flow hood (or a clean surface away from drafts or excessive dust) using aseptic techniques. Lipids should be added last to prevent destabilization of the emulsion in acidic solutions. Parenteral solutions are an excellent media for growth of bacteria and ideally should be used within 24 to 48 hours of preparation. Before use they should be kept in a dark, cool area away from direct sunlight to minimize degradation and loss of vitamins (when these have been added to the solution). Because PN solutions are hyperosmolar, delivery through a central venous or jugular catheter is recommended. Because of the increased risk of sepsis associated with parenteral feeding, a separate catheter or portal should be designated for PN only. Catheter placement and line maintenance should be performed using strict aseptic technique with all lines changed every 24 hours. An infusion pump is recommended to ensure that the rate of infusion is consistent. We generally start with an infusion rate targeting approximately 25% of the calculated goal. If blood glucose concentrations are within reference ranges, then the rate can be increased by an additional 25% every 4 to 8 hours.

Complications Associated with Parenteral Nutrition

Hyperglycemia both at admission and during hospitalization has been associated with an increased risk of complications including infections and renal failure, longer hospital stays, and reduced survival in humans and horses with critical illness or injury.[37–39]

Although extrapolation to a different species with different underlying diseases should always be performed cautiously, it would seem prudent to try to maintain blood glucose concentrations within or close to normal range. In cases in which hyperglycemia persists, the use of insulin infusions is recommended to attempt to normalize the blood glucose concentration (**Box 4**).

Lipid infusions have been associated with allergic reactions, hyperlipidemia, alterations in liver function, and fat embolism. The risk of fat embolization is higher in larger droplet emulsions or in emulsions that have been stored too long and have begun to destabilize. Although solutions containing lipids are useful in providing additional calories, their use needs to be determined on a case-by-case basis. Lipids should be avoided in patients with a predisposition to or pre-existing hyperlipidemia or underlying liver dysfunction. Thrombocytopenia, coagulopathy, fat embolization, thrombocytopenia, coagulopathies, and alterations in cellular immunity are reported with lipid infusions. Triglyceride levels and platelet counts should be monitored regularly when lipids are added to PN solutions.

Box 4
Insulin therapy in response to hyperglycemia

Constant rate infusion: 0.0125 to 0.05 U/kg/h

For a 50-kg foal = 0.0625 to 2.5 U/h

Must maintain on a dextrose infusion to prevent hypoglycemia.

Titrate rate to maintain euglycemia.

Additional complications reported with PN include hyperammonemia and elevations in serum urea nitrogen level from excess protein catabolism, hypercapnia caused by excess carbohydrate metabolism, thrombophlebitis caused by hypertonicity and pulmonary embolism (thought to be caused by destabilized lipid emulsions), and sepsis.[30,34,39,40,41]

Monitoring

It is recommended to monitor blood glucose at least every 4 to 6 hours when starting PN and to adjust the rate to try to maintain blood glucose within or close to the established normal ranges. In addition, daily assessment should include serum electrolytes, venous partial pressure of CO_2, blood urea nitrogen, triglycerides, and ammonia and liver function during the acclimation period. If possible, the horse should be weighed daily. Once a steady state has been reached, the frequency of blood monitoring can be decreased; however, the same approach should be used when discontinuing PN.

Once a patient begins readily ingest and tolerate a reasonable amount of food (25% normal intake or more), PN can be gradually discontinued. Decreasing the supplement by 25% every 4 to 8 hours is generally well tolerated. Frequent monitoring of blood glucose levels during withdrawal (every 4 hours) is warranted, particularly in foals because of the risk of transient hypoglycemia.

SUMMARY

It is clear that nutritional support is an important adjunct to medical therapy in the sick, injured, or debilitated equine patient. What is not clear is the optimal route, composition, or amounts of support. The enteral route should be chosen whenever possible to maximize the benefits to the gastrointestinal tract as well as the patient as a whole. Complete or partial PN is most useful as a bridge during recovery and transition to enteral feeding in the horse. Although the exact caloric requirement for sick, debilitated horses is unknown, estimates are available to use as a target for nutritional supplementation. Research in humans and laboratory animals suggests that even a little nutritional support is beneficial, and the reader is encouraged to consider nutritional support whether enteral or parenteral in any anorexic, chronically debilitated, or sick equine patient.

REFERENCES

1. Hill GL. Understanding protein energy malnutrition. In: Disorders of nutrition and metabolism in clinical surgery. Understanding and management. London: Churchill Livingstone; 1992. p. 71–83.
2. Romijn JA. Substrate metabolism in the metabolic response to injury. Proc Nutr Soc 2000;59:447–9.
3. Powell-Tuck J. Nutritional interventions in critical illness. Proc Nutr Soc 2007;66: 16–24.

4. Gunst J, Van denBerghe G. Parenteral nutrition in the critically ill. Curr Opin Crit Care 2017;23:149–58.
5. Yeh DD, Cropano C, Quraishi SA, et al. Implementation of an aggressive enteral nutrition protocol and the effect on clinical outcomes. Nutr Clin Prac 2017;32: 175–81.
6. Ingels C, Vanhorebeek MEng I, Van den Berghe G. Glucose homeostasis, nutrition and infections during critical illness. Clin Micro Infect 2017;24(1):10–5.
7. Martindale RG, McClave SA, Vanek VW, et al. Guidelines for the provision and assessment of nutrition support therapy in the adult critically ill patient: Society of Critical care Medicine and American Society for Parenteral and Enteral Nutrition: executive summary. Crit Care Med 2009;37:1757.
8. Hoffer LJ, Bistrian BR. Nutrition in critical illness: a current conundrum. F1000Res 2016;5:2531 [eCollection 2016].
9. Stapleton RD, Jones N, Heyland DK. Feeding critically ill patients: what is the optimal amount of energy? Crit Care Med 2007;35(supplement):535–40.
10. Burrin DG, Stoll B, Jiang R, et al. Minimal enteral nutrient requirements for intestinal growth in neonatal piglets: how much is enough? Am J Clin Nutr 2000;71: 1603–10.
11. Hernandez G, Velasco N, Wainstein C, et al. Gut mucosal atrophy after a short enteral fasting period in critically ill patients. J Crit Care 1999;14:73–7.
12. Paradis MR. Nutrition and indirect calorimetry in neonatal foals, In Proceedings of 19th Annual Veterinary Medical Forum of the American College of Veterinary Internal Medicine, Denver (CO); 2001. p. 245–7.
13. Oftedal OT, Hintz HF, Schryver HF. Lactation in the horse: milk composition and intake by foals. J Nutr 1983;113:2196–206.
14. Cerra FB, Rios Benitez M, Blackburn GL, et al. Applied Nutrition in ICU patients: a consensus statement of the American College of Chest Physicians. Chest 1997; 111:769–78.
15. Lacey JM, Wilmore DW. Is glutamine a conditionally essential amino acid? Nutr Rev 1990;48:297–309.
16. Novak F, Heyland DK, Avenell A, et al. Glutamine supplementation in serious illness: a systematic review of the evidence. Crit Care Med 2002;30:2022–9.
17. Rotting AK, Freeman DE, Constable PD, et al. Effects of phenylbutazone, indomethacine, prostaglandin E2, butyrate, and glutamine on restitution of oxidant-injured right dorsal colon of horses in vitro. Am J Vet Res 2004;65:1589–95.
18. Potenza MA, Nacci C, Mitolo-Chieppa D, et al. Immunoregulatory effects of L-arginine and therapeutical implications. Curr Drug Targets Immune Endocr Metabol Disord 2001;1:67–77.
19. Ruth E. The impact of L-arginine-nitric oxide metabolism on ischemia/reperfusion injury. Curr Opin Clin Nutr Metab Care 1998;1:97–9.
20. Scheppach W. Effects of short chain fatty acids on gut morphology and function. Gut 1994;35(supplement):S35–8.
21. Golenz MR, Knight DA, Yvorchuk-St Jean KE. Use of a human enteral feeding preparation for treatment of hyperlipemia and nutritional support during healing of an esophageal laceration in a miniature horse. J Am Vet Med Assoc 1992; 200:951–3.
22. Hallebeek JM, Beynen AC. A preliminary report on a fat-free diet formula for nasogastric enteral administration as treatment for hyperlipaemia in ponies. Vet Q 2001;23:201–5.
23. Hardy J. Nutritional support and nursing care of the adult horse in intensive care. Clin Tech Eq Prac 2003;2:193–8.

24. Sweeney RW, Hansen TO. Use of a liquid diet as the sole source of nutrition in six dysphagic horses and as a dietary supplement in seven hypophagic horses. J Am Vet Med Assoc 1990;197:1030–2.
25. Hansen TO, White NA, Kemp DT. Total parenteral nutrition in four healthy adult horses. Am J Vet Res 1988;49:122–4.
26. Naylor JM, Freeman DE, Kronfeld DS. Alimentation of hypophagic horses. Comp Contin Educ Pract Vet 1984;6:S93–9.
27. Coenen M. Digestibility and precaecal passage of a special diet in dependence on the route of application (spontaneous oral feed intake vs. tube feeding as liquid diet suspended in water.). J Anim Physiol Anim Nutr 1986;56:104–7.
28. Peter JV, Moran JL, Phillips-Hughes J. A meta analysis of treatment outcomes of early enteral versus early parenteral nutrition in hospitalized patients. Crit Care Med 2005;33:260–1.
29. Gramlich L, Kichian K, Pinilla J, et al. Does enteral nutrition compared to parenteral nutrition result in better outcomes in critically ill adult patients? A systematic review of the literature. Nutr 2004;20:843–8.
30. Durham AE, Phillips TJ, Walmsley JP, et al. Study of the clinical effects of postoperative parenteral nutrition in 15 horses. Vet Rec 2003;153:493–8.
31. Durham AE. Clinical application of PN in 5 ponies and 1 donkey in the treatment of hyperlipaemia. Vet Rec 2006;158:159–64.
32. Greatorex JC. Intravenous nutrition in the treatment of tetanus in horses. Vet Rec 1975;97:21.
33. Hoffer RE, Barber SM, Kallfelz FA, et al. Esophageal patch grafting as a treatment for esophageal stricture in a horse. J Am Vet Med Assoc 1977;171:350–4.
34. Lopes MA, White NA. Parenteral nutrition for horses with gastrointestinal disease: a retrospective study of 79 cases. Eq Vet J 2002;34:250–7.
35. Marinella MA. Refeeding syndrome and hypophosphatemia. J Intensive Care Med 2005;20:155–9.
36. Ralston SL. Clinical nutrition of adult horses. Vet Clin North Am Equine Pract 1990; 6:339–54.
37. Capes SE, Hunt D, Malmberg K, et al. Stress hyperglycaemia and increased risk of death after myocardial infarction in patients with and without diabetes: a systematic overview. Lancet 2000;355:773–8.
38. Johnston K, Holcombe SJ, Hauptman JG. Plasma lactate as a predictor of colonic viability and survival after 360 degrees volvulus of the ascending colon in horses. Vet Surg 2007;36:563–7.
39. Durham AE, Phillips TJ, Walmsley JP, et al. Nutritional and clinicopathological effects of post operative parenteral nutrition following small intestinal resection and anastomosis in the mature horse. Eq Vet J 2004;36:390–6.
40. Jeejeebhoy KN. Total parenteral nutrition: potion or poison? Am J Clin Nutr 2001; 74:160–3.
41. Sternberg JA, Rohovsky SA, Blackburn GL, et al. Total parenteral nutrition for the critically ill patient. In: Shoemaker WC, Ayres SM, Grenvick A, et al, editors. Textbook of critical care. 4th edition. Philadelphia: WB Saunders; 2000. p. 898–908.

Moving?

Make sure your subscription moves with you!

To notify us of your new address, find your **Clinics Account Number** (located on your mailing label above your name), and contact customer service at:

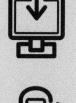

Email: journalscustomerservice-usa@elsevier.com

800-654-2452 (subscribers in the U.S. & Canada)
314-447-8871 (subscribers outside of the U.S. & Canada)

Fax number: 314-447-8029

Elsevier Health Sciences Division
Subscription Customer Service
3251 Riverport Lane
Maryland Heights, MO 63043

*To ensure uninterrupted delivery of your subscription, please notify us at least 4 weeks in advance of move.

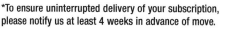
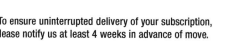

Printed and bound by CPI Group (UK) Ltd, Croydon, CR0 4YY

03/10/2024

01040393-0017